MW01484410

Learning Disabilities and Success

A 20 Year Follow-Up

Here's to all of your successes & to the support you have given me

with love
Mary Ellen

Mary Ellen Clancy

Mackerel Press
2019

Copyright © 2019 Mary Ellen Clancy
ISBN 978-0-9689251-1-9 (paper)

Published by

Mackerel Press
No.2864 HW 245
Maryvale, Nova Scotia, Canada, B2G 2L1

Cover design by Ruth Young, Antigonish, Nova Scotia

Printed in Canada

Table of Contents

Acknowledgments

My first words of thanks must go to the six people with learning disabilities who contributed their experiences and insights. They provide us with a window into the successes and struggles of adult living and learning. I treasure the opportunity they have given me to follow their lives beyond university and the rich source of information and encouragement they provide for the readers of this book. I have learned many valuable lessons from them and from the students and colleagues I have worked with over my years at St. Francis Xavier University. I am grateful for the companionship and inspiration of the many students, friends and colleagues who have explored with me the complexities of education and success with a difference. Their interest in joining the discussion and believing in the possibilities of success helped immeasurably in crafting this study of success. Jeanette Lewis encouraged me to put these ideas into a book not just once but twice. Rod and Brigid Janssen saw the first manuscript and offered their professional expertise on the details of making it happen.

Getting our news into print has sometimes seemed an impossible challenge to me. Certainly the details of this process were unknown territory. Many thanks to Louise Gadbois and Len Macdonald who patiently helped me find the way. Once again Linda MacDonald took the voices on tapes and transcribed them to text with the same careful touch I remember. Ruth Young gave a new look to the cover design that Louise Gadbois created for Education with a Difference. The wizardry of Marcy Baker rescued the formatting process at a crucial time.

To Peter, I owe a debt of gratitude that I will gladly take a lifetime to repay. Here's to the joy of learning and to the people who give us love and hope on the paths to success.

Preface

At first glance, it is hard to imagine a successful life for a person who has difficulty processing information and does not read or write or spell very well. It seems especially challenging when you consider how much we rely on print to communicate our ideas in the learning and working environments around us. How could we expect someone with a learning disability to succeed? One of the significant barriers is the lack of positive expectations for the future. Would you expect to see an individual with a learning disability writing a thesis, earning a post-graduate degree, becoming a teacher, raising a family, leading a multinational seminar, running an e-business, working as a librarian or a chief executive officer? All of these kinds of successes can be realities for people with learning disabilities. This book offers the chance to look beyond deficits and see how success is possible.

This is not a how-to manual in the traditional sense but it is a book filled with hard won insights and thoughtful comments about living with a learning disability. In these pages, we have the luxury of following six adults with learning disabilities beyond their school years. They show us how varied problem-solving styles can pull them forward through adversities and open opportunities in education and in employment. We see the details of their daily lives and how their strategies for accommodation evolve as they mature. Their reflections on the past and their hopes for the future are explored as well as their views on helping and supporting people with learning disabilities.

In an earlier study, *Education with a Difference* (2001), these participants presented us with their insiders' views of the lessons they learned from their successes at university and the critical incidents in their student lives. This book is a sequel to that project and continues our conversations some twenty years later. Those same people are now entering their forties. The chance to take a second look at the progress of their lives beyond university was appealing to us all. It seemed an excellent way to make a further contribution to the discussion of adult success. We have continued the tradition of using pseudonyms. Although the interviews are not presented verbatim, we all agree that the spirit of the conversations remains.

Once again, I have been far from a detached reporter. I have known all of my collaborators over the course of their university studies and beyond. This has allowed an openness and depth of discussion that might not have been possible otherwise. I was counsellor, advocate, colleague and friend to them all. This level of familiarity also allows me to include my own perspective, first as a university counsellor, working to understand and support the development of success strategies and later as an interviewer revisiting my collaborators.

This book is divided into six parts. Each of our contributors has one of the first five parts. Every part begins with a chapter from the university years, as it appeared in *Education with a Difference*. This is followed by a chapter on life at forty, that explores building a career and finding a place in the wider world. Taken together, the two sets of interviews presented here allow us to speak with confidence about the ways that skills and strategies developed in educational settings can be transferred to success in employment and participation in community and family life. The final part contains my observations on what I have learned working alongside people with learning disabilities. There is also a description of the program of support that helped our contributors build their success strategies. This is followed by a discussion of ways to educate the wider community. Each chapter is self-contained, so the reading can be enjoyed in whatever sequence best matches your interests. You can follow the development of each individual or focus on the topic of education or employment.

The insights here are not just for people with learning disabilities. There are also valuable lessons on the complex process of providing effective interventions and building good working partnerships. Together we have seen how education makes a difference beyond the years in school. Hopefully, our experiences will lead more people to embrace a view that looks beyond the obstacles that come with a learning disability to the possibilities for success. Ways of learning and working may be different but as you will see, the successes that life can offer are still within reach. Our goal is to provide a clearer understanding of what success looks like in the lives of people with learning disabilities as they discover the strengths and struggles that make it happen.

Gathering and working with these conversations has been an exciting and rewarding process for me. It is both humbling and reassuring to see what works and what doesn't when you try to be helpful. Following the lives of these young people to see what happened next has provided me with the opportunity of examining my own practice as a professional. I am indebted to them for all of the things they have taught me about learning and success. I am delighted and inspired by their strengths and accomplishments. My challenge in the pages that follow is to pass along the things we have learned.

1

Introduction

How are we to understand what the future holds for people with learning disabilities? Words like "disability" and "learning difference" are not automatically associated with success and yet today you will find students with learning disabilities among the graduates of any high school and post-secondary educational institution. Sometimes we hear of the outstanding careers and achievements of people with learning disabilities and the non-traditional routes that can bring success. Other times we hear discouraging statistics of anti-social behaviour, mental health and physical health issues and a general failure to thrive as independent adults. How do people with learning disabilities excel in education or in employment? Can they find their share of happiness and success as independent adults?

Early on, educators hoped that learning disabilities would disappear as students aged. Educational systems might present difficulties for persons with disabilities but they would also provide instruction. They would offer feedback to measure progress and specialists to assist with the development of learning and advocacy strategies. The disabilities would either be successfully remediated or cease to be an issue once the student no longer had to meet the challenges of a classroom environment. Now we understand that learning disabilities don't disappear when school ends or with the awarding of a diploma. Time and experience have shown that learning disabilities persist inside and outside of the classroom. All too often it is the programs of support that disappear.

Researchers and educators have long been fascinated by the combination of academic strength and weakness that students with learning disabilities present. There has been a recognition of the extraordinary achievements of the few, but there was not a great deal of optimism generally about the chances of success in formal studies, particularly at the post-secondary level. (Brinkerhoff, Shaw & MacGuire 1993) Faced with this prognosis, students with learning disabilities and their families began looking for improvements in programming and support for educational opportunities that would lead beyond high school and into a career that matched strengths and interests. Their advocacy efforts, in partnership with educators and researchers, brought changes in attitude, policy and services that began to allow students with learning disabilities to pursue post-secondary education in increasing numbers.

The gains made over the years are undeniable. There is much to celebrate since the 1990s when our contributors enrolled in university. Acceptance of difference and participation by people with disabilities has much wider cultural support today. Advances in technology have offered accessible options for handling a learning deficit that fit with current trends in using and transmitting information. Speaking and listening to your computer is common place. Sharing an image on your phone can communicate your news. Texting does not require formal grammatical or spelling rules. Websites, blogs, videos and podcasts on the internet can give access to both personal experiences and current academic research results. Optimism about brain plasticity and improving information processing skills has re-emerged. Educators know more about how and when to intervene with programs and supports. Variations on universal instructional design and advances in programming continue to appear. Home and school partnerships are encouraged. There is more information and discussion about the social and emotional impact of learning disabilities outside the classroom and across the lifespan. Issues of career choice and employment are getting more attention. At conferences on learning disabilities you will find individuals with learning disabilities are no longer only the subject of discussion, they participate as consumers, parents, teachers and academic researchers.

In the light of such impressive progress, it seems there is a bright new world for people with learning disabilities. Perhaps if you were a person with a learning disability you would wonder how this list of positives is related to your daily life. Clearly, there are many reasons for optimism but that does not mean that the daily challenges of making your way in the world have disappeared. Despite the progress made, the diagnosis of a learning disability can still be the beginning of an overwhelming obstacle course. It often isn't easy to be different and learn to handle your deficits. Expectations for success in education and employment are still in doubt. We have seen the positive impact that intervention and support programs can have in education but funding for services continues to be difficult for all ages. Programs of support for adults with disabilities are in short supply. There is still much to be done.

Many times I have heard critics ask, "What is the point of pampering students with all of those accommodations for their learning disabilities when they won't have those luxuries in the real world? Who would hire them? How would they manage if they did get a job?" We all wonder about these questions, especially people with learning disabilities themselves. What happens next is a story seldom heard and one well worth telling. Will the strategies students have mastered to become effective learners and contributors work for them outside of an educational setting? It's hard to follow the paths taken or even to define success once young people step beyond the tracks they leave in formal educational systems. Graduates move into a wider world where there are more and different challenges and fewer avenues and systems of support. Can they expect to be out there with other adults leading healthy, independent lives, buying stuff they fancy and making positive contributions in their careers and communities? Or will the realities of a learning disability be a barrier to meeting the milestones that mark adult success?

It is in response to these questions and challenges that we offer the experiences and reflections of six adults with learning disabilities, accompanied by comments from a mentor. Finding success is not just about the resilience of the individual or the access to adaptive technology. It doesn't happen all at once and pathways will differ. But viewing oneself as an able participant is the common goal. Finding success is a lifetime process and we can see it here in the day to day choices that are made. These in-depth profiles allow us to see the complex interplay between the factors that lead to success. In providing them we hope to make the ways to success clearer for others and easier to find.

Who are People with Learning Disabilities?

Common wisdom tells us that humans are a diverse group. We all have strengths and weaknesses within us. People with learning disabilities have very dramatic differences between their strengths and weaknesses as learners. They can excel in some areas and fail to meet even minimal expectations in others. They are full of surprises. Perhaps they can discuss astrophysics but cannot relay a phone message accurately. They cannot catch a ball, but they can tell you the statistics on all the best teams in baseball. They can quote the dialogue from a favourite movie but they have never finished reading a book. They work their way to the top in their job but they struggle to fill in a form or keep track of their house keys. They make brilliant and insightful comments but they stumble with the routines of daily living. These discrepancies are very hard to understand and to live with.

Too often people with learning disabilities are seen as lazy, stubborn or stupid. Perhaps they don't follow even simple instructions. Sometimes they are full of energy and ideas but they can't seem to get assignments completed. Their written work may be brief, disorganized and messy but they can talk their way into and out of all kinds of situations. They fail the easy tasks and solve the problems that no one else can. When flashes of ability appear, this can mistakenly be regarded as proof that lack of effort and motivation are the only problems to be faced. Many times learning seems to be a frustrating and elusive task. Other times they can be excellent mentors or project leaders. Their strengths may allow them to function well enough to get by, but their weaknesses prevent them from fully expressing their knowledge and mask the tremendous amount of effort they have expended for sometimes average results. Some days and some situations are better than others. Variability seems to be the only constant. Although variability is common to us all, it is the permanence, the intensity and the pattern of difference that makes people with learning disabilities stand apart.

Most people can call to mind someone whose behavior matches elements of this description but the definition of the term "learning disability" has been debated ever since the first published attempt was made by Sam Kirk in 1963 (Wong 1998). There are still many thorny issues surrounding the naming and diagnosis of this hidden disability although recent research has done much to clarify the biological basis of the condition. Disputes over financial support and reasonable accommodations often add fire to the discussions. Others resent the stigmatizing implications of the label. Rather than becoming entangled in this debate, I offer a working definition to establish a common ground for understanding our narrators. This is an old favourite with students because of the simple language. It covers the main points and it is easy to use in explaining their learning situation.

> *A learning disability is a permanent disorder that creates difficulties in taking in, retaining and/or expressing information. It usually shows up as a noticeable lack in one or more academic skills in a person of average or above average intelligence. It also may affect one's ability to organize, to manage time and sometimes to get along well socially. It is not to be confused with any other*

disabling condition such as emotional disturbance, developmental delay, social or economic deprivation or sensory-motor disabilities. There is no single profile of a learning disability. Its many characteristics combine in a variety of ways that affect each individual differently. (Learning Disabilities Magazine 1987)

All of our contributors would fit this definition. They have had formal assessments by educational and medical experts at some point in their learning careers to officially document and describe their learning style. They all have significant discrepancies between their learning strengths and weaknesses which are powerful enough to affect their basic literacy skills and achievements.

Who are our Contributors?
Here six adults with learning disabilities reflect on their successes and struggles, first as students in their twenties graduating from university and then once again in their forties. Their varied strengths and weaknesses, both as people and as learners, illustrate the diversity covered by the diagnosis of learning disabilities. They share a commitment to education and a strong desire to succeed, even though they had all been told they would be lucky to graduate from high school. None of these individuals or their families accepted the limitations that the conventional wisdom of the day had seen for them.

Their determination to continue their educational success led them to enroll in the small Maritime university where I worked as a counsellor in student services. There they found an educational setting with a tradition of concern for social justice and community development. Small classes and excellence in teaching was a point of pride. What it did not have was a policy or a program to recognize and support students with disabilities. It is not surprising that these students felt they were working against the odds and taking on a very big challenge. We worked together as they faced the barriers in their new environment and we also worked together to make that environment more informed and welcoming for students with disabilities. They shared the keys to their success with others as part of our Speakers' Bureau and educated the students and professors around them by being successful participants academically and in the wider community.

Succeeding at university was a triumph and an important milestone for them and their families but many questions remained about their future. Facing the wider world as independent contributing adults seemed an even bigger challenge, one which alternately motivated and worried them. Would their success continue as they began establishing themselves as independent adults? How could they manage the new and diverse demands they would face?

Twenty years have passed since those first interviews. Happily, the course of my life and theirs has allowed me to ask those questions and offer their accounts from university days paired with the details of their lives at forty. The two sets of interviews allow us an insiders' perspective on navigating the barriers they faced in the worlds of school and work. They help us learn more about the meaning of a life-long disability.

Defining Adult Success

We all recognize the comfort of feeling successful in our own eyes and in the eyes of others. A personal best or a dream come true can be a great win, but what are the other indicators we might use to look at the success of adults with learning disabilities? Once again we are faced with many definitions. The literature and research around individual growth and development typically looks at measures that demonstrate the ability to be independent and self-supporting. Often studies focus on financial outcomes of salary, tax paying, home and car ownership and include levels of education, stability of employment and engagement in relationships with family and community. Some studies address the issues of negative adjustment by searching public records for reports of violent behavior, criminal convictions and contact with mental and physical health care professionals. Others examine the ability to deal with stress and adjust to change.

These are yardsticks that have not always brought good news to people who are dealing with learning disabilities. Often clouding these results is the reality that people with learning disabilities cannot simply follow along with others and expect to succeed according to established norms. Their successes may be hidden in the standardized timing and points of comparison. Sometimes the very fact of their success and the lack of necessity to disclose their disability make them disappear into the mainstream.

To provide a clearer picture, this book is based on an interview approach. It searches out the ways that the individual differences, which are at the core of a learning disability, can be linked with success in education, employment and quality of adult living. In the pages that follow, our contributors tell how they found ways to use their differences as tools for success. They discuss their struggles and their wins at important points in their lives. They offer insider's views on the complex art of living as adults with a learning disabilities. We believe that a detailed follow-up look at independent living and working life, across nearly twenty years, is a valuable addition to the discussions of adult success. We hope to encourage others to see opportunities beyond the barriers that difference imposes, and create more positive expectations and possibilities for success.

References

Brinkerhoff, L.C., Shaw, S.F., and McGuire, J.M. 1993. *Promoting Postsecondary Education for Students with Learning Disabilities: A Handbook for Practitioners.* Austin: PRO-ED Inc.

Wong, Bernice Y.L. 1998. *Learning About Learning Disabilities*, 2nd ed., San Diego: Academic Press.

2
CHRIS JORDAN
University Years

The proudest day of my life was the day I graduated from university. I had done something that many people had told me was impossible. I felt that this accomplishment was not only for me, but also for the people who had believed in me along the way. I was especially happy because I knew what this meant for my family. Graduating answered a lot of my own questions about my ability and put to rest a lot of other people's doubts about my potential. It made people look at my ability, not my disability. People still might have their own perceptions about my intelligence level, but I did not fail out of university. In that way I think I demystified the idea of a learning disability. I had proven to people that I was smart and I was a success. I was not shut out of education. On the contrary, I was a candidate for social work school. I had choices and possibilities for the future. That was one of the greatest gifts that I have ever been given.

I came to university knowing that I had a learning disability. Every time I sit down to read, I am keenly aware of it. I see things in an inverted order. At times I tend to scramble up the words. For the word "was" I may see "saw". Although my reading speed has increased drastically over my time at university, I still tend to read slowly. I do a lot of memorizing of the vocabulary that I need to recognize in the material that I'm reading. For example, I may need to know the word "constituency". I'll memorize the way that word looks. Once I'm familiar with the terms in the material, my reading ability increases. If words with a similar form appear, like "constituency" and "constitution", I get jarred. I have to be really careful because the meanings are often quite different. Spatial arrangement and the use of fancy types of print can throw me off. To this day I have a tough time reading a menu. Slowing down and staying calm always seems to help both my reading speed and my comprehension. The way I process print makes both reading and writing a difficulty, but you know, I can work around it.

The feelings that I had on graduation day were light years away from how I felt when I started university. I came not knowing whether I would make it or not. I was taking a shot in the dark. If I could do it, great. If I couldn't, it would just confirm all the negative things I'd already been told about my ability and my potential. Past experiences in secondary school had been very detrimental to my confidence. It had been one bad term after another. I hadn't had a lot of great experiences in the school system and very little success prior to grade twelve.

My parents were definitely on my side. I never doubted that. They did all that they could to help me get through the school system. My parents knew something was wrong by the time I was six. With the support of the family doctor, I had been referred to the provincial children's centre for assessment. By the age of eight, I was diagnosed as dyslexic. The testing suggested I had strong academic ability, but I needed a good remedial program to build my literacy skills, and accommodation to allow me to express my ability.

My literacy skills did improve over time, but in the day to day it was hard going. In the early years I had remedial help at school. My parents hired tutors and helped me with my homework themselves. The provincial center was a long distance away, so I didn't have a lot of educators paving the way for me and helping me to develop coping skills. It was a struggle to get any accommodation at all for exams and assignments from my classroom teachers. My mother always had to advocate for me with the school and the school board. Sometimes it seemed more like battling than advocacy. In the last year of high school, I was finally allowed to write my exams in a private room. It seemed as if I was always either in class, with a tutor, or doing my homework. School was a huge struggle and it consumed all of my time.

By the end of high school my confidence level was low and I was very nervous. I needed to be reassured on a regular basis that I could do academic work, but I did have the grades to qualify for university entrance. I knew I would need encouragement and support to succeed at university, but I had no clear picture of how that would happen. In spite of all of that, I still wanted to try university. Much to my relief, things got better at university. Gradually I figured out what I could do and what I couldn't. With some good experiences my confidence grew, but that didn't happen right away. My initial year was filled with anxiety and crisis.

Surviving the Stress
Probably the worst part of first year for me was writing exams. I was very stressed with the uncertainty of the whole year, but exams were the worst. Written exams were a strong, strong wall for me. To this day exams can be a stumbling block, but over the course of the

years I have learned to cope much better with written evaluation. Then I dealt with it the best I could, but it was a very nerve-wracking experience. I would get so nervous and stressed that I would go days without eating. I couldn't sleep properly. I think I made myself sick with worry. At one point I became so physically ill that I had to be hospitalized. I know it was stress-related. There was no other reason. It wasn't healthy for me to feel that much stress because of academics. I see that now, but at the time I didn't. I got through it. I'm glad I stuck it out because now, seven years and two degrees later, I have experienced a lot of success.

Another big source of stress for me during first year was going to speak to the professors about my learning differences. There was a huge amount of anxiety around those discussions for me. There probably was for both parties, but I didn't know that at the time. Nothing was ever just cut and dried for me the way it was for other students. It seemed so much easier for them. All they had to do was go and write their exams at the time and place posted on the master list. Then they got their marks back. I had to go and negotiate with each of my professors for each of my exams. I had to make arrangements for a suitable place, time limit and type of testing, as well as agreement on proctoring and delivery of the exam. I developed important skills that I still use today, but at that point I didn't feel like I was building advocacy skills and managing my learning style. I was just experiencing a mass of anxiety around approaching professors.

Much of my ability to talk about my learning disability has come through my experiences at university. I knew that I had to learn to go and speak on my own behalf, but having the confidence to do it was another matter. I have developed that confidence, but at first it was terrifying. Think about it. I was eighteen years old. I had a low self-esteem and I was insecure about my academic ability. I was in a new environment. I had to approach people who I felt were godly. These were people who had gone all the way to the Ph.D level with their education, and I was asking them to tailor the format of testing and evaluating my work to suit my learning style.

Normal students, or even students who are told that they are above average, would never think of going in at the first of the year to question the format of a course. All of a sudden here I was, not so much by choice but for the sake of my own success, having to meet and negotiate with professors. I had to go to professors and say, "Look, I have this learning difference, a disability." I had to wait while the stunned look on their faces passed as they started to figure out what I was saying. I would explain about learning disabilities and my situation. I could see some professors trying to figure out if I was feeding them a line, or trying to decide if they could tailor things for one person. It was a very intimidating situation.

Many of the professors did not have a lot of knowledge about learning disabilities. I think sometimes I educated them about the topic. At that point I thought, "These are professors. They have Ph.Ds and are well educated. Why don't they know anything about learning differences?" Looking back, I think I was probably the first glimpse they had ever had of an actual person with a learning disability. They might have heard of the concept, but here I was standing in their office asking them to figure out what to do with a real person at university with a learning disability. That was frustrating for me. It was time consuming and it was scary.

I think it took many years, maybe even until my senior year, before I was starting to feel a little bit more confident to make that initial approach. Partly I think that confidence came with an increasing sense of my own credibility. That first year I didn't really know what I could do, or exactly what to expect. All I had was encouragement and backup from my counsellor.

As the years went on, the professors got to know me and I got to know them. They saw me in the class setting. My attendance was always good. I am articulate and I speak out in class. They could always tell that I knew the issues in the course and that I was keeping up on things. It makes negotiating a lot easier. The flip side is that you have to watch your image. You have to get to class and do your homework, no matter how much time it takes. You cannot wait until later in the year to approach the professor. The earlier in the year you can get in there and start advocating for yourself, the better it is. You need to give the professor an understanding of how you learn, and get a feeling for the attitude and approach the professor will be taking.

Some of the bad experiences I've had with professors have happened when I have been too intimidated to go in early and start talking. Somehow I would try to believe that I might be able to get away without any special accommodation from the professor. I would let the term go on and speak with the professor only after I had failed something, or had a problem with a due date. It just made negotiating harder. I would feel much worse because I knew that it was my responsibility to discuss the situation. When the professor pointed this out, I would feel like I was inconsiderate, instead of someone with a reasonable request. Putting it off only made it into a bigger stumbling block. That first visit is something that just has to be done sooner rather than later no matter how stressed it makes you feel.

The Social Side of University Life

One of the other big worries for me was the social component of university. Sometimes when people plan for university, they just look at the academic side of learning differences and neglect the social impacts. When I came to university, I had a low self-esteem, as I have mentioned, but not just academically. Secondary school was full of bad experiences for me, social and academic. I wasn't the type of student who was an all-around popular guy. I had a few close friends, but I didn't get to socialize with many kids. I was always studying. Because I was the kid that stood out in an academic way, I also stood out in a social way and I don't mean in a positive social way. I was afraid this would happen at university too.

I was extremely nervous about coming to this new situation. I didn't know if I would fit in well with other students my own age. I rather suspected I would not. I was thinking, "Will I be the retarded kid?" I don't even like to use the word retarded, but that's what I was thinking. "Will I be singled out in class? Will people know that I am stupid and that I can't do this?" I didn't want anybody to know that I had a learning disability. There were a few people that I had to tell, but the more secretive I could be about it the better. These are things that I don't believe today, but at that point I thought, "God, what am I doing? How will I make it? I don't want anyone to know!"

Not only was I worried that I wouldn't have a social life, but I was also worried about what would happen if I did have a social life. I wouldn't be able to do the amount of work necessary to pass my courses. My parents were worried that if I lived in a dorm with people my own age, I wouldn't be able to concentrate. We all knew that I needed a quiet place to do my work and a lot of time to study. They felt that a roommate, partying and everything that comes along with a residence environment would be too much for me. We decided it would be best for me to live alone. I got an apartment near the campus. It was an experience I can't say that I regret, but it was pretty scary all the same.

Living all on my own was a very big step. I was eighteen years old. I had never lived alone. In fact, I think I had lived a sheltered life in many ways. I had experienced a lot of blows with my learning difference, so I think my parents tried to give me a protected home life to make up for that. They adjusted their life style to suit me. At home I didn't really have to even think about taking care of myself.

All of a sudden I was totally by myself in this apartment. I think it was good because of my unique learning style. It definitely gave me the space and time that I needed to focus on my studies, but I can't actually say that it was something I would recommend for other people. There were times that I really resented being there by myself even though it gave me privacy. Sometimes I felt like I was in prison. I lived by myself all for the good of my education. I guess for academics I was willing to compromise and miss some of the other experiences I could have had in first year. Sometimes I wondered, "What have I ever done to deserve this?" I don't know if someone else would have stuck it out. Everybody's tolerance level is different.

After my first year, I moved into a single room in residence and gave myself a better chance to socialize. By then I knew how to find a quiet place on campus. I knew I wanted to make friends and get more involved in campus life. I knew that I had to have more than just school work in my life, otherwise the stress would be too much. Living in residence worked out very well. It was convenient for meals, classes and the library. I met new people, played intramural sports and just generally got more involved. Socially I was able to relax and enjoy my time at university.

In fact, it was at university that I finally realized I was not all alone. I actually experienced peer support. This was entirely new for me. For many years I hadn't wanted to be associated with learning disabilities. I think many people don't identify their difficulties because of the social stigma. In high school I hadn't known anyone with a learning disability, but at university I realized there were a lot of people in my situation. The students with disabilities would meet, usually informally, but sometimes we had formal meetings. It wasn't compulsory. You could come if you were interested and when you had the time. It was very reassuring to know that other students had experiences similar to mine. It normalized things. I started to feel that I was no longer the only one, but part of a bigger group with other people who were also at university. When I met some of the graduates and heard of their success, it was music to my ears.

Each year we held a transition workshop for high school students with learning disabilities who were interested in coming to university. It was very empowering to be part of that. Being able to show other students what university might be like gave me a sense of my own progress and success. It was one more thing that normalized learning disabilities for me. At each workshop I would meet more people with learning differences who were accomplishing their goals and having their own successes. It was more proof that I didn't ever have to believe those words that used to haunt me, "You're slow. You're not going to get anywhere in this world." I always walked away from those transition weekends with the feeling that learning differences were becoming more recognized and that students with learning disabilities were no longer just being shoved aside. The workshops were an indication to me that there were opportunities for students with learning disabilities to go to university. There was a recognized place for them. It was a great feeling.

A guest speaker at one of those workshops became a really strong role model for me. He still is to this day. We each have a unique learning style. We had similar experiences in secondary school and in our communities. He had graduated from university and was in law school. I saw the successes he had achieved and I really looked up to him. Later I invited him to speak about learning disabilities at a community workshop that I organized. He was an individual who had done extremely well, and continues to do so, under circumstances similar to mine. It was really important for me to see someone not just talking about how to succeed, but doing it. It meant I could too. I latched onto him as a mentor and he became one more driving force for me.

My mentor was very up front about his learning disability. He used to say, "Just because you don't take the freeway, it doesn't mean you're not going to get to your destination. If you have a learning disability, you may have to take a different route, but it doesn't mean you're not going to arrive." I really liked that approach. There are some aspects of my learning disability that have forced me to go in different directions. I have to do some things differently. In that way it has limited me and changed my way of doing things. But that's fine. We are not all alike and our learning styles are not all alike. It doesn't mean that I'm not going to reach my goals. Instead of just trying to convince myself that this was true, it was important for me to see that getting there really was possible.

Managing my Learning Style

With my university courses I spent extra time on the reading and writing parts. I had proofreaders. I probably shared notes and wanted to discuss course material more than most people. I had tutors for the first two years. Sometimes I took a reduced course load. I developed new strategies to become more efficient with my studying time and with the way I produced exams and papers.

In my first year I took a reduced course load. Both the admissions officer and the counsellor had recommended this. I didn't want to feel that I was behind everybody else, so I decided to take four courses over the fall and winter terms, and then finish off the fifth course over the summer. That way I could have a reduced course load, part of the summer off and I would still be able to start my second year with five courses completed just like everyone else. In hindsight, I see what an excellent decision that was. I think that the course relief made a world of difference. There was so much uncertainty and anxiety for me already in my first year that four courses fit very well. To me it felt like a full course load. Some days it was more than enough to handle. I gradually worked my way up to a five-course load. I felt secure knowing that if the load was too much, I could drop back and use the summer to keep up the program pace. Reduced course load was a good option to have.

The availability of technology is a wonderful gift for students with learning disabilities. I found both the computer and the dicta-phone helped a lot for assignments and exams. It's just another world when you can get typed copies of your work. I wish I had learned to use a computer earlier. The spell check and the correcting features were a blessing for me. I used to be so perfectionistic that I would go through agony and stacks of paper trying to get my paperwork to look right. I could not tolerate seeing the mistakes I made in writing things out. With the computer I could make changes easily and take breaks when I got frustrated or tired. I could simply save and walk away. I could print a hard copy whenever I wanted to see on paper what I had written.

Examinations were the biggest challenge for me. I needed accommodations to be able to show what I had learned. I started out using extended time and a private setting. Later I tried other kinds of adjustments. Sometimes I took an oral exam in the professor's office. Other times I used the dicta-phone or my computer. Sometimes I arranged to do a take-home exam. It depended on the course and the professor. It was a learning process. I've had some really good experiences working with professors. Most of the time I got suitable accommodation but sometimes I felt I didn't receive the adjustments that would allow me to show what I had learned. Would I have done as well as I thought possible in those cases? That's a question I'm left with.

At times I would feel uncomfortable about having special arrangements for my exams. Sometimes other students would suggest I was getting an unfair advantage, especially if I was doing really well in the course. They didn't understand that for me writing an exam among two hundred students in a gymnasium just wasn't possible. Well, it was possible, but I wouldn't have been able to write anything sensible.

When I would write an exam on my own with a proctor, my anxiety level would diminish. I was more relaxed. My reading was better and I could write what I knew. If I felt anxious or my attention span was reaching the outer limit, I could get up and walk around. I could just set things aside, take a breather, and then come back and refocus. I couldn't do that in a room full of other students. Later when I was using a dicta-phone or my computer, it would have been even more impossible to do my exam with a large group.

One of my professors pointed out to me that I could write his exam in two hours, or I could write it in three hours, but if I hadn't prepared and I didn't have the knowledge base, another hour wasn't going to make any difference. That statement made me realize that I wasn't there to be tested on how fast I could read and write. The point was to see if I had the knowledge or not. The format of evaluation and the environment of the testing is important to me, but the point is still the same, to show what I have learned. I still work on my writing skills and my test-taking skills. I want to improve, but working on those skills for me involves more than just writing words on paper with a pen. I am trying to improve my ability to use tools, like the dicta-phone and the computer, and to manage my stress. That's what "writing" involves for me.

A Strong Desire to be Educated

I had ability and determination coming to university. I was willing to work hard and make sacrifices for my education. I was used to that. I had a lot of motivation to succeed, but my previous experiences had left me anxious and unsure, and lacking many of the coping skills that I needed to succeed. The ability to do what I did came from me but one of the most important factors for me at university was the support services. The various types of accommodations and the counselling services made an impact on me in a really positive way. The potential to succeed was there, but the circumstances could have easily swayed things in a less positive direction. If I had not had that support, I'm not sure how my future would look now. Time has shown me that with accommodation and support I can soar, but I didn't come to university knowing that.

When I look back at that first year now, I am surprised that I would stick it out. I don't know where that came from. I don't know if it is associated with my learning difference, or if it is just a personal, innate thing. Sometimes I wondered if physically I would be able to do it, but in the midst of all those difficult circumstances, I never did feel like giving up. An education was something that I really knew I wanted. I was willing to do what I had to do to get it. It had never been easy for me. First year was only one example of the things I readily compromised for the sake of obtaining my education. I simply had a strong desire to be educated.

I knew I was in this for the long haul. In the short run I felt uncertain. I didn't know if I would make it at university but I saw university as a stepping stone to something else. I wanted a professional occupation. I was interested in being a lawyer or a public relations manager. After some of my summer jobs I began to like the idea of social work. I enjoyed my courses in political science and sociology. Whatever I was going to do, I knew that I needed more than one degree to qualify for the kind of job that I wanted. The thought that I would be a professional gave me a long-term goal. It was a way of looking beyond the daily grind. It was something to look forward to. It was a driving force.

I have to admit that for my initial degree, another big motivator was the thought of proving to other people that I could succeed at university. So many people had doubted my potential to go to university that the need to show them that I was smart enough to graduate pushed me on. Sure part of it was for myself, but a large part of not giving up was to prove those doubters wrong. Some might say that accomplishing my degree was done with the wrong intentions, or for the wrong reasons. So be it. I don't think it absorbed me and it wasn't the only reason I was there. It worked. It got me through and motivated me when I wanted to give up. I don't think I ever seriously thought of giving up, but there certainly were points when I felt so tired that I didn't know if I could go on. Physically, my body took a lot of beatings over the four years, just from the stress of struggling. I would say to myself, "No, I can't give up. I'm going to do this. I have to do this. It's not just for me. I have to show them that I am intelligent." The need to prove something to those doubters served a purpose for sure.

Keys to Success

I never reached a point at university where I totally gave up, but when I hit a lull, much like any other student, I needed to get encouragement. I really feel strongly that with some of the lows I hit I needed somebody there to say to me, "This is not the end of the world. You can get through this. You have the potential." Today I can answer those questions myself, but at that point, I firmly believe, I couldn't. The potential for my success was there at that time, just as it is today, but the key is the believing.

What I believed at that point could have been very detrimental to everything I was working so hard to achieve. It could have meant the difference between staying or leaving. Having those services there to refresh my belief in the possibility of success made all the difference, even in the brief lulls. Counselling enabled me to refocus and I could not have refocused at that point if I didn't have help. I know that there may be some students who can accomplish their goals without special services. I think that's great. However, I also know that at that point, I just didn't have the coping skills or the advocating skills that I needed. They have developed, but at that point I just didn't have them.

As important as the support services at university were to me, they never turned into a dependency. Now, having had social work training myself, I'm even more impressed with the way they were structured and handled to avoid this. There were services there when I needed them, but I never lost sight of my own goals or my own aspirations. I didn't have the feeling that someone else had taken over for me and done things for me so that I didn't deserve my degree.

I grew up at university. I grew socially, academically and especially in the sense of getting a better grasp of my learning disability. Of course, this is an on-going process. It continues to happen. Learning difference isn't only an academic issue. I will have a learning disability for the rest of my life. How I cope with it and how I accommodate for it are things that I will always have to work out. The fact that the disability will be there is a reality. It isn't going away. As soon as I came to grips with the fact that there was no quick fix, I became more relaxed. I know it is part of me like someone who wears glasses. That's who I am. It's not the end of the world.

Just as my learning disability has become part of me, so have the skills that I have learned to cope with it. When I came to university I knew how to survive, but there is a firm difference between surviving and coping. When you are a survivor it serves a purpose. It keeps you going. But sometimes there comes a point where you can't survive anymore. Surviving absorbs your being. It takes your soul. The first year at university that's what I was doing, surviving. All I knew was how to survive. Just to get through passing was fine. I was satisfied with that, but then I learned how to cope. I learned ways of accommodating my learning style and I learned advocacy skills. I had successes. I didn't have to lose myself in the process. It's all instilled in me now. It's second nature. Those skills will be part of me for the rest of my life and they are definitely the key to my success.

My experience at social work school is a perfect illustration. The social work program suited my learning style even more than my undergraduate courses. My marks turned into As. I became a scholarship student. Even so, one of my greatest fears in going on clinical placement was how to handle the paper work. I was very aware of the responsibility of my internship. This wasn't like doing a paper for grades. I was dealing with real people. I was going to be reading medical files and making notations that someone else was going to have to read. For the first time in a number of years, I felt that anxiety again. The fear was really strong and I was asking myself if I could do it. I kept thinking, "This is it. It's over. I'm not going to be able to do this."

But I'd been through this before. I realized that I just had to go a little bit slower. I had to put in a little bit more time reading and doing notations. Maybe it took an extra hour, but I could do it. One of the great things about the technological advances in our society is that computers and dicta-phones are common now. Everyone in the clinic used a dicta-phone for their notation. I was already an expert. I would dictate my notes and the secretaries would type them up, just as they did for everyone. Since I was a student, my work was reviewed quite often and never once was I criticized for my clarity, or my ability to express what had gone on in a counselling session. That was a wonderful experience. Here I was in the kind of setting where I wanted to work and there was no stumbling block. I had the ability and the means to express it right there along with everyone else. I did well. I got great feedback on my reports and my anxiety dissipated.

The idea of moving out into the real world and looking for work can be pretty intimidating. At times the nervousness I feel about this can be overwhelming. "Sure, I have coped in the academic realm, but what about the real world of work. Will I be able to cope there?" Then I remind myself that I have learned things that are going to be important when I am in the work force. The coping skills that I learned at university got me through. They are life skills. I will have them with me for the rest of my life. I was able to succeed in an academic world that was totally geared for non-learning-disabled students. I was able to get an education in a system not set up for me. Better yet, I was able to do well. I developed multiple skills that saw me through. If I can do that, then I think I can be crafty enough and creative enough to do well in the work sector. My success can continue. It doesn't need to end here. I know it doesn't end here. I have faith.

Lessons Learned

My learning difference is never going to go away. It's there. It's part of me. That's a given. It's how I cope with it and how I work around it that I can change. What if paraplegics decided they didn't want to use a wheelchair and a ramp or whatever accommodation they may need? They would obviously make their whole life a lot more limited and difficult. It doesn't mean that the wheelchair is their whole being. There is no reason that the wheelchair and the lift have to define them. It is enabling, even if it makes you different. Refusing the aid doesn't make the disability go away. It makes you disabled.

I don't use a wheel-chair, but I use other forms of accommodation for my disability. It makes me different sometimes, but I don't see it as a limitation or something abnormal anymore. I guess that's the wonderful thing that's happened to me. It's just part of my life and how I do things. Other people may have a problem with it, but I don't anymore. I think that is an important battle to win. If you can't be comfortable with yourself, and you can't accept your differences, it becomes very hard not to be swayed by other people's views of what a disability is and what it isn't.

Now I never walk away from the term 'learning disability'. I do have a learning disability, but I tend to use the term learning difference. I have become very keen on political correctness. That's my personal choice. I think for me disability is not a word that suggests inability in every fashion, but for many individuals it does. When I say the word disability the initial perception is limitation, not ability. The interpretation is all encompassing. People think of you as unable in every way, shape and form. I obviously don't believe that. I think I'm proof that disability doesn't mean unable. Over the past few years, I've been using the term 'learning difference' to make that point.

My learning disability means that I may have to do things differently. That may be a limitation depending on the situation. It's changed my way of doing things, but we're not all alike, and our learning styles are not all alike. I'm comfortable with that now. It's like wearing a pair of glasses. Sometimes I even forget it's there. The words learning disability don't make me uncomfortable, but I think it makes other people uncomfortable. I tailor my terms for the general public so that they won't think immediately of limitations and inability. It's been my way of demystifying learning disabilities, and communicating who I am and what my abilities are. Explaining all of this used to be terrifying to me. Now it just comes naturally.

As far as helping students succeed at university is concerned, I liked the kind of support program that I experienced. I was able to express my abilities and there was not such a focus on disability. I think that having accommodations available like taped texts and extended times for assignments and exams are essential. Technological supports like the dictaphone and computers are important too. Perhaps the most important thing is to have a person to work with both students and educators to make them aware of the issues and the possibilities of learning differences. Until educators become aware, there is just so much water being treaded. Someone can drown in the process. That person loses an education and not because of lack of ability. Some young individual, who might have the potential to do well, slips away with no education because of uncertainty and lack of knowledge on the part of the educator and the constraints of a system that doesn't allow or promote different ways of teaching and testing.

What would I want for other students with learning differences? My learning difference has pushed me to look at myself and the world. It has changed my attitude. I wouldn't say it has made me a better person, but I think it has made me a more understanding person. I understand that the world is not all painted in one shade. Students are going to have strengths and weaknesses. We are not all strong in the same area. That doesn't mean that we're not capable, or that we're not intelligent enough to do well. I've learned this from my personal experiences. I wish the school system took that more into account. I think too often students who aren't strong in the expected ways at school are dismissed and told that they don't have any abilities. They aren't allowed to express their abilities and work on their strengths. I really feel that's an injustice. That's limiting students, not educating them and to me education is the key to success.

THE VIEW FROM OUTSIDE

I did not really expect Chris to make it through his first year at university. He had intelligence, determination and support from his family, but his anxiety level was so high that I did not see how he could possibly endure the stress he was experiencing and do any coherent work at all. Motivation and perseverance were obvious strengths, but anxiety led him to the limit of his endurance and health. During his time at university, Chris built the confidence and the skills, both socially and academically, to overcome the anxiety that threatened to cripple the expression of his abilities and his enjoyment of life. His story vividly illustrates the interaction of stress, self-acceptance and success. This is how it looked to me.

In his first year at university, Chris was extremely secretive and embarrassed about his learning needs. He was not confident in his ability to do university level work and it was his fear of failure that drove him to disclose his learning disability at the counselling centre before he started classes. The admissions officer had helped him make contact with me. Chris knew that he would need accommodation for his learning style and support for his transition from home. In spite of his reluctance to expose his vulnerability, Chris was willing to do whatever was necessary to make sure that he had a chance to succeed.

Setting up the mechanics of his support system, although it wasn't easy, did not seem to be a major problem. Chris worked well with his tutors and his professors. He appeared to have no trouble finding notetakers on his own. It was the prospect of evaluation that made him panic. As his anxiety rose before a test or an assignment deadline, he would photocopy more and read less. He would arrange and rearrange his support schedule and his priorities. It seemed to be the only thing he could do. As the piles of unread material grew higher, he would become more and more stressed. It was painful to watch. There seemed to be no way to calm him so that he could actually study.

Through all of this panic, Chris always managed to look great in the latest designer clothes. He had his own apartment near the campus. He carried a briefcase and was fond of taking taxis instead of walking. He showed all of the signs of wanting and enjoying a fine lifestyle. To an outsider, he looked fine. However, from my point of view it looked as if he was engaged in a colossal misdirection of his resources and attention. He seemed focused on appearances rather than the underlying realities of his situation. What I did not realize then was that Chris used this style to cope with the pressure he felt to look and be able. It was part of how he was trying to convince himself and the outside world that he could succeed. Chris looked very different once he had gained confidence in himself and earned his academic credentials. He waved goodbye to me wearing overalls. All of his possessions were in a hockey bag, and he was ready to set out on his own to find work half way across the country.

As his counsellor that first year, I was not sure that I was getting through to him at all. His fear and lack of confidence seemed to be overwhelming. His tutors felt the same way. We all admired his persistence and the courage it must have taken to keep on trying under the stress he was experiencing. It simply did not seem possible to get him to try different strategies and come to easier terms with himself in his new learning situation. I was so distracted by his anxiety that I didn't realize the extent to which he was listening, nor did I give him credit for the new things he was trying. We watched helplessly from the sidelines as he drove himself to exhaustion. It seemed clear that he felt out there all alone, trying as hard as he could. I listened and encouraged him when I could. We were all pleasantly surprised when he returned the next September with very respectable marks and another course completed at summer school.

Surprising people and beating the odds was really nothing new to Chris. In his initial clinical diagnosis at age eight, there was concern about further deterioration in his neurological processing and mixed views about his ability to succeed in school. His future looked very uncertain at that point. There were few resources in his community to help meet his particular educational needs. His parents advocated for him and he was able to use effectively the encouragement and remediation that was available to him. No one would deny that it was a major triumph for him just to get to university. He certainly was not planning to quit once he had made it that far, no matter what the cost.

Chris was used to functioning without an extensive institutional support system for his learning disability, but social and emotional supports were essential for him to do what he needed to do to succeed. In spite of his overwhelming anxiety, it seemed to me that Chris was able to persevere through his first year on sheer determination and the encouragement offered by his parents.

When Chris arrived to begin his second year of studies, it was clear that something quite remarkable had happened over the summer. He came back to university ready to be a student with a disability. Not only had his personal approach changed, but Chris was also ready to educate the community about learning disabilities. He started to make plans for a panel of speakers who would put on a workshop at the university for educators, students and parents. He had set this goal for himself after his marks had arrived. Remembering the previous year, I was concerned that he was taking on too much and said so. This did not deter Chris. He enlisted the support of key people all the way up to the president of the university. He convinced speakers to come along and a large audience to attend. The entire event was a huge success. The outcome of Chris's time at university never seemed to be in doubt after that. Certainly there were rough patches and crises of various sorts, but they never really sent his anxiety skyrocketing again. His beliefs about himself and what he could accomplish had clearly changed.

Chris completely changed his social style too. Instead of hiding away in his off-campus apartment, studying to the point of exhaustion, he became involved in campus life. He moved into residence and played house league sports. He found new friends and mentors. Eventually, he even managed to get himself thrown out of the campus pub for rowdy behaviour, but only once. He found the courage to try new strategies for studying and exams. He could hear and use feedback in a more effective way. He became more independent as a student and as a person, although it still required a huge amount of energy for him to complete each year. It was an amazing transformation.

Chris developed into an effective self-advocate and a valued member of our Speakers Bureau for community education. He was a founding member of our support group for students with disabilities and I knew that I could always count on him to be part of our transition workshop for high school students. There he worked his way up from peer facilitator to keynote speaker. His pleasure at being able to develop and maintain a supportive network of friends and teachers was as obvious as his determination to change the way the world regards people with learning disabilities. He is a volunteer board member for the Learning Disabilities Association of Canada and his research on students with learning disabilities in Nova Scotia has recently been published. He continues to believe in the importance of educating systems and communities about learning differences. From his own experiences, he understands how important an informed and consenting environment can be for a learner.

I have heard Chris say that at university he learned that with accommodation and support he could soar. I believe him. I saw it happen and it was a very exciting process to watch. His optimism about his future success shines through in his comments. It is an optimism that I share.

3
CHRIS JORDAN
World of Work

I met with Chris in an historic office building in the heart of our capital city. This seemed the perfect environment for someone who has always been fascinated by politics. Through his network of contacts Chris had arranged a setting for our discussion that was easy for me to find, private and offered a beautiful view of the city. He had thought of everything. He hasn't lost his warm and friendly manner or his ability to get things done. Chris is very capable and accomplished. It shows when you meet him. He looked every bit the executive in the midst of a busy weekend. He also conveyed his appreciation of the time we would be spending together and his enthusiasm for the goals of the project. The stage was perfectly set for him to share his reflections on learning disabilities and success. Here they are!

Success: I can make it look easy but it's not

If you consider that my grade school teachers expected I was headed for a life on social assistance, I have built a surprisingly successful career. It hasn't been easy. Every day it's a struggle but the struggle is more palatable with the skills I have. Going into the world, I know I can cope. Even though I am no longer in an academic setting, I still use the strategies and negotiating skills that I learned at university. I have better coping skills today and I have accumulated successes but I don't take anything for granted. It's not like, "Ok, now I've reached this point and I'm not learning disabled anymore." That's just not true. No matter what, my disability is not going away. I have a life-long learning disability that is not just related to academics. It's not like having something that will change after university. In fact, in many ways it gets tougher.

I think the whole idea of a learning disability has many facets to it. There's the career and family aspects as well as the educational ones. There's the emotional impact and the impact on self- esteem. All of this has become more real to me over the years. Now I know what lifelong disability means in a way I didn't seventeen years ago. Back then this was more of a theoretical idea than an experiential understanding. Today I have lots of experiences to make that fact real to me.

I don't want to sound like a wet blanket. To be honest I do not feel sorry for myself. I don't want you to think that everything in my whole life is smoke and mirrors and struggle. I have a family, a house and a good job with a good salary. Back home twenty years ago no one thought I would be up to much. I have pushed myself to do things in life and I have succeeded. Everyone is driven for different reasons. As I am always saying, there's nothing wrong with being driven, but it does take a toll in stress and anxiety. I'm sure lots of other people feel like this too but for different reasons.

Snapshots from Life after University

After I qualified as a social worker, I put all my belongings in a hockey bag and headed out West with a one- way ticket. I had one hundred and twenty-six dollars in my pocket and some friends to stay with until I found work. When I tell that story now, I can't believe I did it. I had earned a Bachelor of Arts degree in Political Science and one in Social Work. I wanted to see where they could take me. I hoped this would be the next step on my way to a professional career.

I was supposed to go to Calgary for six months. I went just to test it out and I ended up being there for ten plus years. I didn't have a fixed job waiting and I couldn't find anyone to hire me for what seemed like a long time. After five months of looking I couldn't get a professional job. I decided I would give it one more month and then I would have to pack up and go back East. In that final month, I was offered a position as a social worker at a First Nation's reserve in the North. I knew it would be a big challenge but I've always been up for challenges. For me everything is a risk and everything is a new adventure. I always thought, "Well okay, I'll take a chance. I'll try it." Growing up knowing that I was different, I learned that nothing comes easy. Besides I didn't want to go back home empty handed so I took the job.

I probably got that position because I was new and eager to break in to the profession. They had a lot of problems in the community at the time and it sounds like they still do. I worked there for a couple of years. The turnover of social workers was very high. The locals told me when I started that every month there was a going-away party because people were leaving so frequently. All the same, it was a good experience for me. It was definitely an eye-opener and a growth opportunity for sure.

When I left there, I was promoted to being a case work supervisor. I guess I was rewarded because I had stayed as long as I did in a very tough spot. It was definitely tough. I became a supervisor for the provincial government in Children's Aid for a number of years and worked my way up to being a regional manager. In the middle of all that I took two leaves of absence. One was to direct a community program and another was a secondment back to a troubled First Nation's reserve. As I said, I am always interested in new challenges.

I began to feel that I needed further education to keep moving forward in my career. When my supervisor at Children's Aid asked me what my long-term career goals were, I decided I'd like to be in administration rather than staying with clinical work. If I wanted to be an executive, he suggested I try a Masters of Public Administration (MPA) or a Masters of Business Administration (MBA). The current trends in social work seemed to favour those degrees for an administrator and either would allow me more job flexibility than a further social work degree. In the end, I applied to do an MBA in the Maritimes. It seemed like a good chance to build some new skills and go back closer to my family at the same time.

While all of this career progress was taking place, my personal life had changed too. I met a wonderful woman and we married. When I was accepted into the MBA program, I moved with her to Halifax to begin that degree. In the end, we stayed in Halifax for only one year. I wound up doing the rest of that degree part-time, so I could resume my job as a regional manager back in the West. We had a daughter that year. That changes your life. When our daughter was one year old, we moved to Ottawa. There was an excellent job opportunity there for my partner that also allowed us to be closer to her family and mine. We still live in Ottawa today.

My first year in Ottawa I took a break from Children's Aid. I worked as a manager with a community health centre on a one-year contract. I applied for the position on a permanent basis but I didn't get it. I had done the job for eleven months with very positive evaluations but I couldn't be hired permanently because I wasn't bilingual. In that job not being bilingual was a deficit I couldn't overcome. I decided I would go back to Children's Aid where I had plenty of experience. I found a nearby county where being bilingual wouldn't be an issue. It meant about an hour commute but it was a good job for me and it allowed me to finish off my MBA.

I worked on that degree over too many years to note. After years of part-time studies, I finally went to my convocation. I'm the only person I know that has done a master's degree program at three different universities, in three different provinces and still graduated from the same program he started in. I became a visiting student wherever we lived. With some negotiations, all these courses were transferrable back to my original university in the Maritimes.

In the middle of all this, with grad school and changing jobs, my partner and I had two more children. I juggled a toddler, a set of twins, going to grad school part-time, and commuting to work full time as a manager of Children's Aid. My partner had a demanding job too. My mom was ill at the time back in Nova Scotia and a lot of the responsibility for dealing with her care and support rested on me. It was an incredibly busy time.

Three years ago, I applied for a job back in Ottawa as executive director for a not-for-profit organization which serves the homeless and the hard-to-house. That's the job I've been doing for the past three years. We serve a lot of people. In addition to counselling we have a Food Bank, an Emergency Drop-In Centre and a program for Learning English as a Second Language.

Getting the Job

Some people with disabilities say that you have to be twice as good as anybody else in order to make it worthwhile for people to select you or to keep you. I know that feeling but the reality is there are essential skills for success in most jobs. There is a standard of performance that is required. If you need to produce material in written form then that's what you have to do. That's where the accommodations come in. You may not do things in the way people might expect but you still have to get them done. There are certain things in my job as an executive director that I have to do. Those requirements have nothing to do with discrimination. They have to do with job performance. If you can't accommodate to reach the necessary standards, you may get the job but you won't keep it.

I have heard the advice about not mentioning a disability until after you are hired and you've signed on the dotted line. I haven't done that and I have still been able to be the successful candidate. I didn't want to be employed by somebody who, if I didn't tell them until after I was hired, told me it was not going to work out. It's similar to the reason you want to identify to the professor at university early on. If you wait until you can't meet a deadline or a performance target, it sounds like you're making an excuse. It almost highlights the issue of weakness rather than showing your competence to deal with the situation.

For my current job, I told them that I was learning disabled. I had two interviews. In the first interview I didn't mention anything about my disability. The second interview was more of a compatibility assessment and that is where I thought I needed to tell them. They asked me the routine question "Is there anything further that we should know about you?" I decided this was the time. They didn't need to know anything about me personally. That was none of their business but I knew my disability could impact my role in the agency. They needed to make a decision knowing about my learning disability. Here I am applying to be the face of the agency and I can't even spell and I can't write a letter without an editor. What would they think if I didn't mention that?

To be hired and then seen as a person who had intentionally withheld something important would not be a good way to begin. I didn't want them worrying I would make the agency suffer. They had to know and understand how things could be managed. I always take this approach but being an executive director was much different than any role I've been in before. The stakes seemed higher and the challenges greater. It's really important to have a good relationship with your board. If you're working at the will of the board, you don't want to be there if you're not in sync. We are three years along in my contract and things have worked out.

Right now, my annual performance evaluation is due. This time, instead of the teacher, it's the chair of the board that assesses my work. I know the things in my performance review where I will not shine are going to be things that relate to my disability. I'm reminded that as much as I try to accommodate and change things to be successful, there is nothing I can do to make my deficits disappear. This evaluation is very important because we are in discussions about extending my contract and a potential remuneration increase. I'm already feeling a certain level of anxiety although things seem to be going well. Will my board continue to value my work? Will they see beyond my disability?

Applying for jobs and having evaluations make me consciously aware of my deficits and the areas where I have to get accommodations. In an academic setting you're expected to perform. If you don't perform, or if you don't come to class, you may fail. It's your problem. In the workforce there's a different kind of expectation about level of performance. You are being paid. People expect performance and it's about more than just you as a person. It's about your productivity. You work for the agency or the company. That's why you are there. You have to produce and if you can't produce, you can't be there. I have never come to a point where I've been about to be dismissed, but there's always that fear factor in the back of my head. Will I be able to do it? I have to do this right or else. I feel that's the reality.

There are other executives out there who don't take two or three times as long to do some things or who don't need the support that I do. I have to work two times harder and spend more time. Since my writing skills aren't so good, I have to be damn articulate. At university I wasn't the best test taker so I had to go to every class and ask a question to make sure the professor knew I was there and keeping up. I had to be seen to be working hard and having good ideas. That doesn't change in the workforce. You can't let your guard down. You have to be hopeful that people are going to be understanding and helpful although your experience has shown you that is not always the case.

I know I should move on in the next twenty-four months for the sake of my career. If I make a change will my next employer be as understanding? If you were hiring people, would you hire the person who is going to need all of this extra support or would you hire the one that doesn't? If you can't write a briefing note on your own, maybe you're not capable enough to be a chief of operations. When I was hired as a new worker twenty years ago, I had to face issues like that. Those fears don't change. In fact, they are probably more real now than they were back then because the stakes are higher and they pay me a lot more money. But you know I have been hired for more than one good professional job.

Getting a Good Match in your Career

I have always been consciously aware that the ability to get accommodation would have an effect on my career path. For me, the time it takes to write and to generate the presentable final product are the biggest challenges in any job. I tend to procrastinate with certain things because it is a struggle. You put me in front of a piece of paper and I can feel my heart start beating. I would rather do anything than be put in front of a piece of paper. It's always like that and I always seem to take on jobs that have lots of paper work including written reports. As a result, I have had to disclose my print difficulties and negotiate accommodations in all of my jobs.

At this stage of my life I feel like I have become accomplished and skilled in many ways. But to be successful in the kind of jobs I want

I've signed on to a life of negotiations. Writing is my big deficit. I can't change that. I can accommodate it. I can support it but I can't make it go away. I'm still so dependent that I can't mail a letter without someone reviewing it. I find that hard in spite of knowing I can negotiate good accommodations. Whatever the demand for paperwork is I have a level of anxiety in any job because of that deficit. I need to be able to make accommodations or I just don't do well. Sometimes I take honeymoons for a minute and just forget about it. But the accommodation has to be as much a part of my routine as any other routine I have. The few times that I haven't done that in my life, I just very quickly go downhill.

Sometimes my anxiety level has been really, really high around dealing with print. I come home and I'm ready to crash or I am already crashing. I've done that more than once over the years. My life partner has pointed out that I'm a sucker for punishment. She asks, "Why don't you find a job that doesn't have so much paperwork?" I don't think about it until she mentions it. I don't know why except that I had this image of myself with a career as a professional. I didn't ever see myself as being someone who would be anything else. Everyone has a different goal but for me it is being an executive in a business suit dressed for success and all that comes with it. To some degree I still hide behind the clothes. I don't think that has changed but it is probably less true now than it was when I was younger. With that image always comes the type of jobs with paper work attached. It's a huge issue for me but you can't have one without the other.

Children's Aid is well known for the importance of documentation in their work and that's where I started out. I could have picked something that was less paper intensive but that was the first professional job on offer. Part of the reason I left Children's Aid was because paper work is a very important part of the job there. So I have made some changes around that requirement. But I've always had jobs and wanted jobs where dealing with written reports was required.

I knew it was a big risk taking on a job as an executive director. I thought, "I want to be an executive director so I have to try it." It was the same with university. There have been lots of times in my life when it was very scary to take on something new but I take the risk anyway. I know my deficits and I knew that my deficits could easily be highlighted in that job. At the executive level you're more vulnerable. You only have a contract for two or three years. If you don't walk the line and make good things happen, you're readily dismissed. It has not been an easy ride these last three years. There have been times when I would just as soon close the books and walk away but I'm not someone who walks away from challenges. That's my point.

Even though I just said that I have had a very difficult time, I think it is difficult for any executive director, not just one who has a disability. You have to learn all of the politics of working for a board of directors and the politics of your team. You can be let go at the will of the board. All of those things you face whether you are learning disabled or not.

I'm in a comfortable place now. My learning disability is not a factor but it is always there. It's easy for me when things are going well to try and forget that I have a learning disability. In many situations, especially if print isn't involved, I can put it behind the scenes. The chair of my board points out that my oral presentations and my written deliverables are two different things but we all agree that I am a good fit here. I've been able to set the tone in the agency. The programs are providing good services with stable funding and everybody there works well with me. The reality is that I can't go to the extreme and say my disability doesn't exist because then the only person in the room I'm kidding is me. Denying my disability makes me disabled. If I didn't have the accommodations and the support network behind me, then I wouldn't get to where I am now.

Challenges of Disclosure

There is always a risk of saying that you're disabled. Once you are something other than what people expected they start making assumptions. It unsettles them. "If you're disabled what does that mean?" That question is even more important when employment is involved. One of the things that I'm learning as I get older is that people admire someone who has a difference and tries to integrate as much as they can into the main stream. If you don't try to single yourself out, people admire you more. I probably didn't know this when I was younger. At the same time, you have to keep the right balance. Some people need to be in the know but if too many people are informed, you start opening up a whole can of doubt about your abilities that doesn't even need to be there. "If you can't write, maybe you can't do a lot of other things. Maybe you shouldn't be here." This stuff still happens.

All through school there were people who told me the only reason I got better marks than they did was because I had unfair advantages. Sometimes I think about the amount of people who made an issue of the fact that I would write an exam in a different room. If they only knew what it was like for me. I didn't set out to get what they called an 'advantage'. I would love to have just gone and written that damn exam with everyone else and left in a timely fashion like they did.

It was no-win for me to discuss grades, especially when they were good. In my university days there were people who were happy to do note-taking for me until I got a better mark than they did. Then they didn't want to be my note-taker anymore. As long as you are equal more or less, it's fine. When you exceed them, you're seen as a threat not someone to be helped. This was a lesson I learned very early in school. It was really clear how some of my fellow students felt and I just didn't want to hear it.

In the workforce, when I was promoted to regional manager over other people who had been very helpful colleagues to me, some of them weren't so helpful once I was their supervisor. As long as I was working in a position below them it was fine. I think there are parallels here with women in the workplace. When I talked to some of my female colleagues who don't have learning disabilities, I found that they have gone through struggles similar to mine. It was okay as long as they were equal to their male colleagues but not if they exceeded them. Things that may have been supported before would be used against them. That's exactly what happened to me when I was promoted.

After I became regional manager it was very obvious that some of my colleagues were trying to put obstacles in front of me. They stopped saying, "we can help you with this." or "don't worry about that!" They knew my weaknesses and they stopped being understanding about them. It wasn't covert. Their true colors started coming out. "How dare you pick the guy with the disability?" No one would say that, but that was the reality they were acting out.

Once you've become more accomplished there's also a way that it's even more difficult to reveal your disability. In a certain sense, it makes it harder to go back to stating that you can't read and write very well without accommodation. People expect you to be competent in everything. They are used to you contributing a lot and being a strong performer. They are surprised and it can be uncomfortable for everyone. I'm still amazed at how true that is.

Today, when I was setting up space for this meeting, I called a friend of mine to make the arrangements. She asked what the meeting was about and I told her I was doing an interview about my learning disability. She was just shocked. She's a really dear friend of mine and we have worked on many projects together. She couldn't believe that I had a learning disability. I could hear the shock in her voice. "Oh! You have a disability?" and I don't know what other things she started thinking. I'm trying to be humble here. I think I've been successful. I've tried my best to do the best with what I have and yet for some people, such as my friend today, it's shocking that I have this disability. What I'm trying to say is that my gift of overcoming my deficits also creates barriers for me.

Now I probably will have some kind of conversation with my friend about my disability. I think she is a very well educated and a very forward-thinking person but sometimes people have only this negative perception of a disability. I don't know yet what she was thinking, but it seemed like she was thinking, "How could you be disabled and be as accomplished as you are?" It does make a difference in the way people treat you once they know you have a disability.

When it comes to supervisors, things are even trickier. Disclosing means you are identifying your vulnerabilities. Throughout my career I've had to adjust to new supervisory styles, like it or not. You don't always get a good match and sometimes when you do there's a change. Some supervisors are easier to negotiate with than others. The one time I didn't explain, it didn't go well. I should have just bucked up and said from the very beginning, "This is my reality. This is what I need." It was just sheer pride on my part and not being humble enough to disclose. I was called in and asked, "Why are you not getting things done in a timely fashion?" I don't think anyone does themselves a favour by not disclosing even though it does present risks.

I have worked with all kinds of supervisors. Some can be helpful and understanding. Some can be sort of indifferent. Or some can be mean-spirited. One of my supervisors who knew my deficits used to poke at my Achilles heel. She would ask me for briefing notes on the spot, even though she knew very well that if I gave her my written notes, they would look like they were written by someone in primary school. With the right supports I could provide her with briefing notes but not "immediately". It was almost as if she was upset with me about other things and used that tactic to draw attention to my weakness. It got to the point that I felt she was doing this to work me out of my job. My stress level was quite high during the time I worked for that supervisor. If you have someone who is not on your side, they know your weaknesses and they can use them against you.

The person I am working for now is just the opposite. She is amazing and she has been very supportive to me. I always get the feeling that her reminders are coming from a point of goodness not malice. She's not by nature a micro-manager at all, but when it comes to written things, she seems to feel that she can take liberties with me. It's an area where she is unsure of my performance. She knows my deficits and she always makes sure that I make the adjustments I need. These are accommodations that we have both agreed to and that she has helped me arrange as part of my workplace support. She can't seem to trust me to follow through on the paper work so she gives me reminders. The difference is that she is very positive about my work and I know she is on my side.

My point is that in an employment setting there are real risks to telling the whole truth and disclosing, but it is usually the best choice. I have to take a leap of faith that people are not going to use my deficits against me because I need accommodations to do my job. In most cases it has worked out that way. A lot depends on the company you keep. If you are in the company of people who want to push your deficit and make it a point of ill will, then your deficits are very intimidating. It is very scary. You start thinking, "I could lose my job if I don't perform in a certain way." In contrast, when someone working with you comes from a point of good will, you can open yourself up to be more vulnerable and more effective.

Negotiating for Accommodations on the Job

For most of my professional career I have had a lot of support from my colleagues and employers. When I have disclosed my disability, they have recognized my abilities and helped me make the adjustments I needed. Without that information they would think I was some kind of slacker. They would be left wondering why does this guy function really well sometimes, but other times he just doesn't. Now as executive director, I have the good fortune to work for a very supportive board of directors. In our office I have people who help me play to my strengths. There is a person whose job was newly created in large part to do my writing. Her job title is manager of communications and community outreach. Along with other duties, she edits my letters and does any big communications that have to go out. My employer was great about arranging this. The whole team is aware of how I work and they accommodate me. Without their support I couldn't do my job.

Even now just thinking about my struggles with paperwork makes me nervous. Well, not exactly nervous but it makes me conscious that I have a deficit. No one wants to dwell on their deficit. But you know the dragon. It can rear its head every once in a while, and I can find the whole process of being helped demeaning. I've had to become more thick-skinned when my insecurity resurfaces. Now when I hand things over, I am prepared. My communications always come back with all these changes. At first this made me really anxious. I'd be in my office alone and I'd be saying to myself, "I'm stupid. I'm just not getting it right". I have to convince myself that it's my own insecurity talking not the reality. I have to say, "My assistant is working in my best interest. This is not about my deficit. This is about sending out the best crafted letter that represents the agency in the best way with my signature on the bottom."

You know, I don't actually give anything out in hand-written form. I would not do that even to my assistants. If there is something that has to be written, even an email, I always send it electronically in draft to either my executive assistant or the manager of communications. They proofread it and send it back to me. Then I cut and paste it into an email and send it off. People have to be on call for me, all of the time. If I indicate that the correspondence has to be out as soon as possible, they are great about it. They will drop whatever they are doing and deal with my work.

Sometimes I find it really frustrating. I would like to be able to deal with writing immediately myself but I can't. I have voice–to-print software in a version that's actually pretty good. It's definitely affordable now. As much as I've tried to get used to using the program, I've never really been successful with it. It seems like one extra step. I've always had to get someone to check things anyway. Maybe it's because I'm just not a technical person and I'm more comfortable with people than machines. The thing is, I have an executive assistant. It comes with the job. If I was a front-line social worker, I wouldn't have those things. Maybe then I would use the software.

I've become less sensitive about this type of support. Other professionals have executive assistants or speech writers who review what they've written or even write letters for them. That sort of second look or editing is not uncommon but because of my history I sometimes leap to something that may not be there. If you are somebody who was critiqued in not such positive way in the past, it's hard to shake those images. It resonates with years of memories of someone looking over my shoulder and second-guessing me. Not even second guessing me but someone who is criticizing and not in a helpful way.

I know I have troubles with organization and managing my time. I have to deal with the fact that I've never really had a sense of how much time it takes to do something. I've had to learn to be more organized and to have people organize me. My assistant does all my scheduling. Every morning she gets me going and helps me plan and get ready for the day. Giving over that power is really hard, especially if you're used to winging it and creating your own schedule. Again, I have to remind myself this is what an assistant expects to do.

I know that I do commit to things in the moment because I want to do it and I aim to please. I always want to say yes, instead of thinking of scheduling and all of the reasons why I should say no. I'll say, "Don't worry, I'll be there." instead of saying, "Let me check first and I'll get back to you." I have all these things on the go plus kids to look after. Sometimes I commit to more than one thing at the same time. I wind up with multiple events and a really complex day. Mostly I can pull it all off.

Even though my life is very busy I still took on a leadership role in a national campaign for five months. I don't regret it though. I couldn't let an opportunity like that pass me by. It was a great experience. I got lots of positive comments on my participation and expanded my network of contacts across the country. That's good for me and good for the agency. Besides, this way I've been forced to learn even more about how long it takes to do various tasks.

Many of my accommodations have come with being a nice guy. I always have to be a nice guy even when I don't feel like it. I feel guilty saying that but the bottom line is that no one wants to help the guy who is a pain. They'll just do the minimum. I have to be cordial with a lot of people even though they are not so cordial back to me. The reality is that people don't go out of their way for people they don't like or they think are not nice. That being said, I have had great supports throughout my career and those people skills that I have developed have had real advantages to me in other ways. There are times when knowing how to negotiate and delegate really pays off. It helps you get all kinds of things done.

Home and Family

Life presents us with different challenges at different stages and raising children marks a new stage in a person's life for sure. I have three small children and I love them dearly. My daughter is nine years old and her brothers are five-year old twins. My life partner and I share their care. A child is something very special. You look at your own children with a love that is very unique and very powerful. I feel my children are my greatest accomplishment.

Sometimes, when my boys are being a bit challenging, I see in them some of the characteristics that I have. They may very well have a learning disability. I don't know. They are only five years old. We'll see where that goes. When they behave in ways similar to the way I behaved when I was young, I find myself impatient with them. While I was watching them early this morning, it was painful to see some of the things they were doing. I know they were not consciously trying to be anything but themselves, but it was still painful to watch them. I now see how some people might have perceived me at that age. I can understand their lack of patience. Maybe those people weren't as mean-spirited as I thought they were.

When I look at my children, I hope they don't have a disability like me. No one wants to be different in that way. I don't want my children to have the life of heart ache that I've had because I was exceptional. I don't want my kids to be holed up studying like I was. I want my kids to go to school and go to university and study but have fun too. I want them to enjoy their life experiences. I don't need to be the noble person and the good example to them. I don't want to be the dad who dies passing on the message, "I've been through a lot and look what I accomplished. This is what you have in store for you." It's not that there's anything wrong with being disabled but it is just so much easier if you are not. Why would you wish that for any child?

As much as I love them, my children present me with one of the biggest challenges I have in my life right now. You might be surprised, but it is reading stories to them. It makes me want to escape. Here I am forty-two years old with nine years of university, two undergraduate degrees, a graduate degree, and relative career success in an executive position. I have made lots of rewarding friends and connections over the years. I just worked as a regional manager in a national political campaign. After I leave here today, I have to go to a function and then I will go home to work on the X million-dollar year-end budget for my board of directors. Yet my biggest intimidation every day is reading a story to my children.

When I sit with my children at the edge of the bed and I feel like I can't read a book that is geared to a five year-old without struggling on the words, it smacks me with the fact that I have a life-long learning disability. In the other parts of my life, I've learned the ways around just being myself. When your brain is wired the way mine is, you always need to find ways to accommodate your deficits. You have to be on your guard and ready with some way to manoeuvre around an obstacle. With my children I don't want to do that. I just want to be with my kids. I want to be sitting on the edge of the bed and be able to read a book to them and not stumble over the words. But I can't. It's my reality and it is not going away.

Their mom is very well read. She loves to read and she loves to read to the kids. Sometimes they read three or four books a night. When you read a children's story there's nothing worse than when it doesn't have a smooth flow. When their mother reads, it's just like watching a movie. It's consistent and relaxing. When I read, I'm stumbling and pausing. When their mom is not available and I have to read to them, my heart just starts beating wildly. I will make every excuse. I will keep them up later so I can tell them it's too late for a story. But they are catching on. They complain "Dad never reads us a story". Their mom, who is a great support, makes an excuse. She knows it's a very emotional situation for me. I said to their mom, "Can they not just have the Jack and Jill books anymore? Do they all have to be chapter books with big words?" We had a laugh but we both know what a huge obstacle this is for me.

Until the time that they could read, I was able to make up the story as I went through. I would ad lib. Now with the nine-year old who reads French and English fluently, it's not the case anymore. I sit down with my boys and my daughter and start reading a story and my nine-year old is correcting me. She is not malicious. She's very bright and a lovely child. She is just pointing out, "Daddy, that's not right." When my daughter was young, I sometimes memorized the books she liked so that I wouldn't stumble. She liked to read her favourites over and over. Now with the boys, I can't do that. They have all of these books that people have given them as gifts and they'll pull them out at random to be read.

Sometimes I get the nine-year old to take the lead on the stories. I tell her that she's such a good reader I would like to have her tell the story. Probably, if I put my mind to it, there are lots more ways that I could manage this. But should I get around it? Is it okay to do that? Is it like cheating? That's where my insecurities resurface. Reading is where I'm most insecure. I'm still obviously somewhat – give me a word – ashamed or embarrassed. When I'm reading to my kids, I'm as real, as core, as they are. It's me. There's no one to help me. There's no one to do anything for me. It's just me and that's a really humbling, embarrassing place to be.

When you are at work, you're on your guard but you have to be. In so many other settings I would have reason to be more intimidated and I'm not because I've mastered those situations. I know how to cope. Friday night I was at a four hour think tank meeting with prominent politicians and people that I grew up watching on television. We were all talking about the art of politics. I'm on my game in that room. I'm working the room and from the emails that I got the next morning I did it pretty well. To sit and read to my kids seems like a basic skill at forty-two years of age, but it is my biggest challenge. My heart is palpitating more walking through that bedroom door than coming into any director's office. I can actually feel myself getting anxious before their bed time because I know I'm going to have to read. They are aware of my difference now and at that moment I don't want to be different.

When I'm with my children and they're in their pajamas and we're all sitting on the bed I want to be able to read a book like their Mom does and not have them looking at me like I'm a dummy. They are my children and you know they are not seeing me that way but that is how I feel. I'm vulnerable there. I know I can work around the reading but the problem is the way I feel. I feel that saying to my kids that I don't read makes me look like I'm stupid. I don't want my kids to know. Sitting on the edge of that bed is more embarrassing and intimidating than waiting to give any speech I might have to make. If I did a public speech where I told that story, I think people there who are learning disabled would say "I know exactly what he is saying."

Emotional Baggage

Even though I was trained in social work, I never really firmly believed in the importance of childhood development until I got older. Now I realize how much of an impact those early years had on the later part of my life. I had a very rocky road early on. I don't think you get away from those scars. I really don't think you do.

I've had to be more responsible than I would have liked to be. I know there were lots of times when I haven't been responsible but for the most part, I've had to be super responsible and that's tiring. You never really get to just have fun. I had to take a good hard look at reality from a very early age or I wouldn't have survived. You don't bring your parents to school. You are on your own. If there were a choice, I would not want to have gone through it. I would have loved to have gone through a relatively flawless childhood. Kids made fun of me, the whole thing. I would have loved to have more friends. I was way too mature, too young. I'm forty-two and I have friends that are fifty-five and older. When I'm in their company, we all feel like peers. I've always had to be older and I resent that. I feel I lost an important part of my childhood. But all of this doesn't mean that I'm paralyzed by insecurity. Obviously, I'm not. The reality is having a learning disability is not a great way to go through the world. It's particularly tough at a very young age. As you get older, you see more of the world and as much as life can be difficult, you begin to see that people are not all the same. There are more different people out there. It's not just you.

When I went to university, I finally sort of fit in somewhere. I could see that there was a place for everybody and it was good to be different. But leading up to that time, I'm amazed at the amount of people who actually get out of high school to get to university instead of blowing their heads off. Maybe things have changed, but what a pressure cooker those years are! The other day I talked to the mom of a young guy with a learning disability. She said every day she worried that she'd come home and find him dead. He was suicidal and had been for some time. I asked her to think what it would be like if she went to work every day where she was an outcast. You know, even though I couldn't do anything to change her situation, I think it helped that she got a way of understanding what it must be like for her son. I think that is the first step in making things better.

I hope people understand that one person's learning disability might be different from another's, but all of us have to cope. Coping doesn't take away the core emotions. For me everything is about strategy. That's my reality until the day I die. Sometimes it makes me resent the fact that I have a disability. Just because I put on a really good face doesn't necessarily mean that at the end of the day, I don't feel insecure about who I am. In the day to day I don't think I ever feel good enough. As they say "Fake it till you make it."

I've had great successes but I still never feel like it is good enough. When I set goals it's more a sense of "I've got to do this." When I achieve something, it is usually followed by a sense of relief that I've gotten through. I remember how proud I was when I graduated from university. I was proud when my children were born. The other times in my life, I don't reach that feeling of peace and contentment. I've had glimpses and I hope for more.

When I look back to my years in high school, I can see that I met with enough success on paper to get to university, but I would have loved to have gone to university and been successful or not successful depending on how hard I worked not on getting proper accommodation. The same things that made me feel insecure back then still make me feel insecure today. When I sign up for an academic course today, I still feel as nervous as I did when I was eighteen. No matter what the situation, I'm always conscious in the back of my mind that I'm one step away from falling. My whole life I have to depend on my colleagues to help me and work with my accommodations. I always have to be on my game to make things go more smoothly and I still feel the need to please more than I should. Those triggers for my insecurity are still with me. I cope and I strategize but at some moments that just seems like the art of bullshit. If I could change it, I would rather not have had a disability.

At one point I worked with this lady who is highly successful and very hard working in a top managerial position. She told me something in confidence that blew me away. She said that her biggest fear was that she might become a bag lady. Today I am still shocked by this. I didn't pursue her reasons but, in her mind, there was a fine line between being at the top of her game and being a bag lady. Yet she is the most hardworking, organized and proficient person I know. Like my friend, I always feel that there is a fine line between me being successful and then not. This is where my spirituality comes in. I comfort myself by believing that there is a reason why a kid from a small town, with an alcoholic father, lots of issues, a severe learning disability and little support from the school and community ended up where I am versus stuck back there. I'm not always as humble as I should be, but every day of my life I never let myself forget that.

My life partner has a saying, "We all have baggage and if you don't have any baggage then you haven't been anywhere." I think that's true. I wish my situation was different in some ways but let's be honest. As much as it's a cliché, I am glad that I had the opportunity to learn from my differences. Well, I wouldn't have minded if my life could have been a fraction less stressful. There has been a cost over these years.

Supporting Success

Being successful has come with measures of support and struggle. I take credit where credit is due. I take credit for the fact that I worked hard all through my education but I don't know how I would have gotten out of high school without my family's support. Then going to university was the biggest challenge I have ever faced. I still feel that way after all these years. I've had lots of experiences that one might see as a big challenge, but my toughest struggle was making the transition from high school to university. It was the greatest leap of faith that I have ever taken in my life, but once I got there it was the most supportive in lots of ways. You know, university is a very consenting environment. That's the irony of it all.

I still think about how grateful I am for the supports that I did get in my undergraduate years. I learned about accommodations that were good options for me and I developed the skills of negotiating to secure them. I was not overly accommodated. I would say that I was appropriately accommodated. If I had been more dependent then, I would have been much more vulnerable now. I was forced, with mentorship, to maximize my potential and do what I needed to do in terms of challenging myself. Had I not taken the steps to go and talk to professors and negotiate for my accommodations myself, I don't know how I would have managed in the workforce. It was better than having things fixed for me. I wasn't left alone by any stretch of the imagination. I had guidance to manage for myself and I always felt I had back up. Being in the Maritimes, we used to joke about the wisdom of the old adage of teaching a person to fish as opposed to feeding them a fish. If I hadn't 'learned to fish' at university I never would have been able to succeed in the rest of my life.

It was a surprise to me when I did my graduate studies that other support programs wanted to do everything for me as they saw fit. They didn't want me negotiating for myself. They didn't value me working with the professor to find out what was appropriate for each particular course. I felt they wanted me to be dependent on the program. I knew the difference from my earlier experiences. I knew how important it is to your success to be able to discuss the course and the options and to learn to advocate for yourself. My point is that if I hadn't learned those skills at university, when would I?

Some of the things I saw as huge struggles in university, now that I am in the work force, they don't seem like so much of a challenge. I guess a lot of people could say this about their own lives. Now I've got more things on my plate and it still takes me twice as long to do them. Where do you get extra time in a busy life? You don't. When I was twenty, I could pull an all-nighter. I can't do that anymore. I've just had to learn to work smarter and advocate for what I need. In school you are young and inexperienced. You can have people who advocate for you. In the workplace, you don't have parents or student services to arrange things. You have to put your pride in your pocket and say "This is my reality and with this accommodation, I can do well here." That's what I have to do at every place I have worked. When you are thirty or forty there's no excuse to avoid it and, for me, no succeeding without it.

I don't see as much understanding of disabilities in the work force as I thought there would be. I thought the education system was a special situation. At university I told myself, "These are the people I'm educating. They weren't expecting someone with a learning disability. I'm trying to teach these professors how to work with me. I'm going to go out into the work force where my strengths are and my learning difference won't be an issue anymore." It wasn't like that. It wasn't that people weren't accommodating but it was probably less support rather than more. People also felt that it was not really their problem. It was mine. Luckily, I am a good negotiator.

Where are the supports for adults with disabilities in the workforce? What if you were somebody who graduated from university and didn't have the good fortune that I have had? Would you end up bailing out because you were perceived to be failing in your job? If you don't have support, you can't shine. I still struggle with that and I'm consciously aware, as much as I want to fall into the fabric of the carpet and not be seen as someone with a disability, there are times when I can't. When I'm confronted with the areas where I have deficits, it comes rushing back in my face that I'm in this difficulty because I have a disability. I start saying to myself, "If I could just write on my own. If only I didn't need to have someone edit what I do." I could go on with examples of my if-only's. It's just not something that as an adult of forty-two years of age I want to have to deal with but there is no leaving it behind. That's the reality. I have a lot of support to get me through times like that. But what about somebody who is out there without that support? Where do they go?

I don't know what legislation there is to protect adults. At one time, I was really involved in the rights and advocacy for students with learning disabilities but I don't know what that means in the workplace. What are the supports that are available or required for people with disabilities? I have been able to negotiate accommodations without having to go to any third party or government agency to advocate on my behalf. I've had the great fortune of having people I work with who've made accommodations for me. But what if you worked for someone where you were denied that support? Could you succeed?

When I went to university there seemed to be a bit of a movement with more students with disabilities going to post-secondary education. I'm still left wondering what happened to those who graduated from university or whatever training institution they picked. I knew people who were trying to become teachers or lawyers or nurses or learn skilled trades. How are they managing through life? Are they falling through a different set of cracks like they were when they were in school? Is there something to be done?

I think there is a bigger discussion to be had about being a person with a learning disability and I think there is an audience who would like to be part of that discussion. If I'm struggling it makes me wonder about other adults with disabilities. Maybe I'm just the sookie in the room. It could be there are lots of people with disabilities doing really well out there, but I wonder if there are. It's hard. I'm just really interested and I hope there will be research to look at where people with learning disabilities are today. There is not just me.

The Strategic Lifestyle

I look back now and I know there were some very hard times, but I guess I just got better at advocacy. I still struggle and I face challenges that make me anxious. It has been years of constantly accommodating my disability. At every stage I've had to negotiate. That has been the consistent theme running through all these years. As I keep saying, a learning disability is not something that goes away. At points in your life you are faced with it. Sometimes it's a surprise but sometimes it's all too familiar. I accommodate and I cope and I do what I need to do. I survive. I've been surviving and getting through things my whole life as far back as I can remember. I want to say it gets easier but it doesn't.

I've had my share of successes and I've had some great times. I've met some wonderful people and some of them because of my disability, but every day is all about strategy. Throughout my adult life I've had to use advocacy skills to make those cold calls and start the conversations about what I needed. When I was part of that national political campaign, I had to call people on the fly and advocate for my candidate. I attribute the success I had in that campaign to those skills I learned back in my undergraduate years to survive. Thankfully, I have those skills of managing and negotiating otherwise I wouldn't have gotten where I am today. I would have given up. I wouldn't have had it in me to keep on trying.

My point in all that is probably not what you might expect me to say. If I had my way, I wouldn't want to have a disability. But the reality is that I do. Some days it seems like I am perpetually coping and constantly strategizing and negotiating. Definitely there is a level of awareness and planning that I need to get me through the day. My partner says I am always acting like the host of the party, not a guest who is there just to enjoy the occasion. I always feel like I have to be ahead of the game. I don't really remember being what people call "relaxed" and I don't know how I would change that. Some things become automatic but there is always something new. Being constantly on your guard is a way of being. It's my way of being, if that makes sense. If you talk to people who are learning disabled, I think you would find that they all constantly need to figure out how to manage. Maybe they don't have to do as much as I do, but I think we all need to be three steps ahead.

There are lots of good things in my life but some parts of it have been very disappointing and stressful. At the same time, there is no two ways about it. I've had a good life. I have a career. I've travelled the world, met a wonderful partner and we have three beautiful children. The life that I've lived was out of necessity versus out of choice. I think that necessity has benefited me in some ways. The important thing is this way of living works and it works well for me. In spite of the level of stress that you have to carry when you operate this way, I'm comfortable with being uncomfortable if that makes sense. I'm comfortable with this driven, push yourself, keep-going style. That part is my choice and I can make it look easy even though it's not.

THE VIEW FROM OUTSIDE

Chris has taken risks and accepted challenges and responsibilities that have earned him an impressive list of accomplishments. He has been able to tame his anxiety and use it as a motivator to find the opportunities that have given him a life filled with successes. He has not allowed his learning disability to be a barrier to his professional ambitions. He is now an effective administrator and a highly skilled negotiator for himself and others. In social work he found an arena where his ability to analyze situations and work in an oral culture were highly valued. He played to his strengths to build his career. He transformed the negotiation and advocacy skills he developed at university to accommodate his disability into career credentials. The type of position he competes for comes with the ready-made accommodation of administrative support. His social skills make him easy to work with and in his various jobs, he seems to be a master of organizing good accommodations and taking care of business. He may have trouble reading print but his ability to read people and situations has allowed him to excel.

Clearly Chris thrives on being busy. He holds down a demanding executive position, cares for his family and does extensive volunteer work in the community. He has found many ways to express his strengths and competencies. Part of the pleasure of his volunteer work is that it allows him to pick activities where he can demonstrate his abilities without the frustration of paperwork. The extra bonus is the many connections and friends he makes. The social awareness and friendly easy way with people that he developed at university have played an important role in his success. When you meet him today it's hard to believe that he was once a lonely isolated soul who did not seem headed for a life filled with successes.

Chris doesn't deny the reality of his accomplishments but the young man who set off from university might be surprised by the difficulties he continues to encounter. In telling his story Chris doesn't allow us to forget that his successes do come at a cost. He makes clear the emotional weight of carrying a lifelong disability. He is constantly on the alert as he searches for ways to transform difficult situations into opportunities. Bridging the gap between his professional skills and his literacy skills is not easy. The discrepancy is painful. It takes a toll on his sense of independence and confidence. He feels the burden and necessity of accommodation and pays a price in stress, anxiety and his own sense of not being good enough. The pain of his deficits remains especially when he simply wants to read to his children.

When confronting his disability Chris is careful to remind himself and the reader of the ways these emotions fuel his career achievements and his strategic life style. He knows he needs to be careful and maintain a balance. His career aspirations have led him to rely on a high degree of workplace accommodation and the support of others. Sometimes this makes him uncomfortable. His deficits with print are a source of stress but he has not chosen to lead a more relaxing life.

He uses his hectic pace and the comfort of his history of success to maintain a fulfilling personal and professional life.

As you might have guessed, Chris hasn't stood still over the time it has taken me to get his reflections into print. He is now the chief executive officer of a national advocacy group. He loves the title, the travel, and the excitement of the big stage. He appreciates having the challenge and opportunity of wrestling with issues of equity and diversity on the national and international scene. He still believes in the power of education and the possibilities of making communities more supportive for people with a difference. The young man who believed that he could soar once he had the tools to accommodate his disability, was right.

4
BOB MACDONALD
University Years

The note on my test said, "Come and see me, Bob. We have to talk." I couldn't understand what the teacher of my law class would want with me. I knew that I hadn't cheated, but I thought I must be in trouble about something. It was October of grade twelve and we'd just had the first test in my law class. It was fill-in-the-blanks and I thought I'd done okay. My grade was in the high sixties and that was about average for me. What could be the problem?

This teacher was one of the few in the school who didn't have a classroom, so I went and found him in his office. What do you suppose he asked me? "Did you ever have a reading test?" That struck me as an odd question. No one had ever raised this with me before and to the best of my knowledge I had never had a special reading test. I can't remember now exactly how he put it, but he suggested that I had a reading disability. The term learning disability was not mentioned. He said he would find a test and see what it would prove. Well JEEZ, that kind of shocked me, but whatever! I waited to see what would happen. For the first time the question had been asked and even though I didn't dwell on it, I wanted to know the answer.

Now this conversation took place in October. Around Christmas I asked him about the reading test and he said he was still looking. He was a teacher, so he couldn't spend one hundred per cent of his time looking for a test for me. Then it was January and he was still searching. He suggested that I watch my spelling and concentrate more. When I asked in March he said, "Well, you know Bob, you have a fairly low-level problem. As long as you keep ahead of it, you'll be fine." When I asked in June, he thought maybe I was just a poor speller. It seems that in the whole of the Nova Scotia school system he could not find this learning test for me. I got a grade of sixty-six for the law class. That year I graduated from high school and never thought anything more about it.

After high school graduation, I floated between wanting to go into engineering or to trade school. I was always under the impression that I would either build bridges or blow them up. I enjoy carpentry and all kinds of construction stuff. I have always been told that I am a great production person. I'm not great at the fine details, but for basic building I never have trouble getting the job done. I was of the opinion that my previous experience would carry me through the uglier problems of trade school. The idea of trying engineering still appealed to me, but I didn't have the proper math courses to qualify for the program.

By September I had decided to take the next steps toward engineering. I took two math classes at night school to meet the admission requirements for engineering and tried out university with some part-time courses. I talked my way into first year engineering courses in graphics and computer science. I chose English as an elective, primarily to get it out of the way. By October I was humming and hawing and wondering if I should speak to my English professor about the possibility that I had a reading problem. Finally I got up the nerve to go and see him. It was my first meeting with him and here I was telling him that I'm in introductory English, but I probably have a reading problem and I need a test. It didn't seem to bother him. He said that he was in his first year of teaching at the university, so he didn't really know the system. However, he would make some calls and get back to me. I waited to see what would happen this time.

Four days later I was beginning my assessment. The professor said that it took him about five phone calls to find the right contact and I was on my way. I had some interviews and I had the testing done. I found that, yes, reading was a problem and there was evidence that I had a learning problem. Well, that sent me into a tail spin! I was just angry. I wouldn't say shattered as much as angry. I kept thinking about how things had been in school before all of this suggestion that I had a reading problem.

It all just kind of hit me after the testing. The law teacher had told me that this was the sort of thing that should have been picked up when I was in grade two. That phrase reminded me of a little incident that had happened in grade two. There was this sentence. It was a fill-in-the-blank sentence that I had to do and I couldn't get it. I couldn't understand the concept of the sentence. It involved the word 'should' and I just didn't understand. I couldn't read that sentence. Still to this day, if you showed me that sentence I probably could not understand what it was trying to say, or what 'should' meant, or anything else about it. It was your classic case of dyslexia. It just didn't make sense to me. The teacher was glaring over at me. The class was over, another class was coming in and the teacher was still glaring at me. The music teacher was starting up with the next class and my teacher was yelling at me to finish this sentence. Finally she threw up her hands in disgust and told me to get out of the classroom. You know,

I still don't know what I did wrong. At the time I just thought, "The teacher doesn't like me. I don't like that teacher and I know a lot of other people who don't like her either."

The thing that kept bothering me was the fact that I never did have a reading test to see if I needed special teachers. There was always some kind of special educator at my school. If someone was falling behind, that person would be taken out during English or math and given a refresher. I remember there were a couple of people in grade one and in grade two who went out with the special teacher. Every year it happened, right up to grade six. It seemed like everybody had a turn, except for me. I never got to go. You see, I slipped through this crack.

Maybe it was because my marks were always average? In class, when I heard information or saw something done, it was nice and straightforward. I understood it. Yet when I went home to study, there was something lacking and I didn't understand one bit. I could always explain things to someone else when they were having a problem, but when it came to the test, I always scored about average. My marks were nothing great, nothing fantastic. I think the teachers felt that I just couldn't be bothered to exert myself. Later when they did those standardized tests for grade achievement and career aptitude, I would score well. I don't know how I could, because they were written tests with lots of reading and multiple-choice answers, but I would always do better on them than in my classroom tests. So I think that kind of tied into this whole thing of why I was just seen as lazy when it came to testing or exams. The comments I got were, "He's obviously not trying" or "He's just too lazy to understand." Still, I never went to one of those resource teachers to find out. Was I lazy? Or did I have a problem?

The other thing that really upset me was an incident with the principal at junior high school. She took me into the hallway and really tuned me out with a speech that went something like this: "Why aren't you doing well? You are just lazy! I'm putting you on probation. You have got to pull your marks up!" It never occurred to her that I might have a learning problem. In her defense, I'd have to say that there wasn't as much known or discussed about learning problems then. I don't know what the adult world thought, but from my perspective, I still question the whole thing. I never saw a special educator and by the time someone raised the idea I was in grade twelve. Then the teacher couldn't find a reading test for me in the whole of the school system. There was something definitely wrong there.

After the testing at university confirmed my learning problems, I was just bitter, evilly bitter, for about six months. The memories of those incidents would flash back into my head. I even wrote that principal a hate letter which I never sent. The letter vented my frustrations. I got it all out into the open. I put the letter away and asked myself, "Where do I go from here?"

For the longest time, I thought that I would just go to trade school. At university I found out that engineering was out of the question. In the engineering and science courses I was always apprehensive. I was just sitting there and I was never sure if I was doing the right thing. I don't even remember the computer course I took. In the engineering graphics course, the professor taught by setting a problem and then having us follow the textbook to work it out. Everyone else would open up the book and just start flying along. I would just sit there. I didn't understand one bit. The second-year students always came in to give us a hand. I would wave over someone I knew and he would explain to me exactly what it said in the book. Then I could understand the problem and do it, but I couldn't understand it until it was told to me. Later I could go back to the book and understand it, but I had to hear it first or it wouldn't sink in. It was the same for physics and calculus the next year. I just couldn't keep up. There weren't enough hours in the day.

After the testing, I began to understand why some of these things were happening. I was trying different ways of dealing with the material, but it wasn't enough. Maybe if I had started using some of these strategies at the high school level I could have gone into engineering, but at this point it was ancient history. The only bright spot was English. I had taken that course to get it over with, but it turned out to be the course that interested me the most. English seemed straightforward to me. It made sense. I wasn't the greatest at it and my grades weren't the best, but I could understand and enjoy it.

By the end of my second year at university I was on academic probation, because my marks in the sciences were extremely low. Trade school was looking like a good idea again. I went to the community college and checked it out. I met the most uncooperative guidance counsellor I have ever run into. He was also the most stressed out. He was impressed that I had been to university, but it looked like the accommodations I needed would just not be there. I had friends who had gone to trade school and, judging from that, I did think that I could get through. My marks might have been a little low in some areas, but overall I think I would have done quite well.

I knew quitting university could be an option that would work out fine. I had friends who went to university and friends who had dropped out to work. One guy is a bush pilot. One guy works on the fishing boats. I think he's off on a trawler near Japan. Another fellow, who was always fascinated with bombs, does survey work for blast testing in the oil fields. They just said, "University is not for me."

But I have never been one of those people who wanders off and is a trail blazer. I am just sort of content where I am. I want to move on in gradual steps. I explain it this way to my friends. If life was a swimming pool, some of you would dive right in. It wouldn't matter to you. You would just be right in there. Me, I like to see if there's water in the swimming pool. I like to see if there's a shallow end and a deep end, and if it has been properly cleaned. Are there life preservers and a life guard who is qualified? If all these factors are in place, I'll stick my toe in and call it a day!

It would have been a huge lifestyle change for me to stop university and go someplace else. I decided to stay at university and study English. I know it seems like an odd choice for someone with a reading problem, but I enjoyed English as well as some of the sociology courses. Besides, my grades were good enough in those courses that I could get off academic probation and continue to study. By this time, I had gone through the assessment process and identified my problems with learning, along with my strengths. I had gone through all of that bitterness and anger, and accepted the idea that I wasn't like everyone else. I knew I had this information processing problem that I couldn't always explain, or even understand myself. What I wanted to do now was figure out how to get around the problem. I chose the road that I wanted and I stayed on it.

How I Learn

I learn best when I hear information and observe people doing things. I love movies. Most of my quotes are from movies. I don't just memorize things. I understand the concept and then associate it with examples. My short-term memory isn't great, but repetition and association really help. Once I have the ideas, they stay with me. I like solving problems whether they are in carpentry or in politics. I can analyze problems and break them down into a sequence for discussion. Precise summaries are my specialty.

What's the problem then? I have trouble dealing with print. Reading, spelling and writing are a problem for me. At university, print is a major part of how you get the information you're studying, and a major part of how you show what you know.

Reading

I have difficulty reading. Now that being said, you know I can read, but I may have difficulty understanding what I have just finished reading. I can read a newspaper quite easily, but when it comes to academic reading at the level of journals and theoretical pieces, it's more difficult for me. I can find anything in the library. I'm good at giving other people a hand with finding a reference, but when it comes to understanding the article, I have to go over the print three or four times before I completely grasp what I have just read. When I read for pleasure, I usually stick to stuff that is fairly straight forward. When reading any passages with a lot of quotations, explanations or descriptions, I usually just read what's in the quotations. When you just read the dialogue, you miss a lot and you have to go back over until you get the full picture.

I was able to overcome this reading barrier by using taped text books from specialized audiotape libraries. When I listen to the text as I follow along in the book, I can understand the material as well as anyone else. It sounds so simple, but the trick is in getting the material in audio form, and finding the time and the machine to play it. But more of that later.

Writing

Writing is also a problem. Spelling is a big part of my writing problem, but punctuation and grammar are also a bit of a mystery. To me, A, E, I, 0 and U are optional letters. They don't have to be used, or I can interchange them. They really have no meaning to me. When I write, I constantly have to be aware of what I'm writing. I have to focus so much on it that I lose out on the content. In class, I can't listen to the content if I'm focusing on taking notes. I'll get hung up on a word like "complexity" and I'll be missing the rest of the idea. My notes end up being half completed with words mis-spelled, which makes them harder for me to read. Then I have to go back over them to figure out what exactly I was writing and what it meant.

To cope with notetaking from lectures, I would get the professor's permission to tape record the class. In the end I wind up spending twice as much time listening to lectures as everyone else. The first time I hear the lecture in class, I relax and listen and take my chicken scratch notes. The next time I hear the tape of the lecture, I use the pause button to think about what was said, or I rewind a section if I can't understand what was going on. It is a lot better than asking a question in class that is way off base. By the time I finish listening and transcribing the notes, they are nice and clear and straightforward. Well, they are clear to me. No one I know can read my hand writing. Cleaned up on the computer, my notes look good. Friends will sometimes ask to borrow them. My typing is fine, but my handwriting just won't do.

Sometimes I had a friend take notes on carbon paper for me as well. We would compare the notes and I could see whether I was staying on track or missing anything. We would also discuss our perspectives on the material. Some professors will lend you their notes. I didn't find that as helpful. The process of listening again to the material and being able to slow the process down to a speed I could manage, was the most beneficial. With my system, I had good notes in the end and I had been over the material so many times that I didn't really need to look at them. I knew the material way better than most people.

It's not just school writing that is a problem for me. Casual writing is the same. When I send letters to my friends, I start out by explaining the rules:

(1) Words that sound the same but have different meanings are interchanged, i.e. "to" could be replaced by "two" or "too."

(2) Any word that I am not sure about will be PRINTED. This does not mean everything written is correct.

(3) I write words the way they sound to me.

(4) My letters never have much point except to ramble on about myself, or complain in general, or at the worst, spread gossip.

(5) My handwriting is very small. When it gets bigger, it has a tendency to become sloppy and even harder to read. In other words, do not be walking down the street and try to read this.

(6) Note: This message will not appear again in later letters so try to keep these points in mind.

This usually gets a laugh and I feel comfortable enough to carry on writing letters in my own way. With professors I have a different approach. When I write papers for courses, I use my computer with the spell check and grammar check, and sometimes a proof reader when I have time. At first, paper writing gave me more trouble. I needed quite a lot of help from an editor or tutor. Now I'm quite independent when it comes to papers. I can even give other people a hand with setting up a research question by breaking down the problem and getting their ideas organized. An eight-page paper seems pretty basic to me now.

In exams, I like to use a dictaphone. That way I get to produce my answers orally, in private. Then they can be typed and given to the professor for marking. Working in a quiet setting helps and I may take extra time. I have to be careful to make sure I have understood the questions. Sometimes I do oral exams if the professors prefer. I'm not good at oral argument. I don't pick things up quickly enough to be able to toss back as complete an answer as I would like, so I always ask for a few moments to get myself organized before I begin. It takes me a while to sort things, but then I am precise and I can get the facts out. Because I learn by understanding the concepts and linking them to examples, rather than just memorizing a list of facts, I am able to show the professors that I know what I'm talking about. Fill-in-the-blanks tests are much harder for me. Retrieving just the right word or phrase is a big challenge. Oddly enough I can do quite well on multiple choice tests, in spite of the reading.

Time Management

Doesn't all of this coping take an incredible amount of time? Yes! I worked hard every day trying to keep up with the class. A chapter of reading was for me an arduous journey. Reading with a taped text can be quite slow. Many times you also need to find a reader for journal articles. Just doing the repetition and having discussions with a classmate takes time. As well as all of that, I was spending easily twice as much time listening to lectures as other students. Then there were papers. I worked evenings, nights and weekends. The best part was that working this way gave me access to the information that everyone else had.

There is no question that one of the biggest barriers was learning how to plan and budget my time. Even after I figured out ways of getting around my learning problems (like taping the lecture, getting a notetaker, finding a tutor or a proof reader, or getting a taped text), it was not that simple. You have to plan ahead, sometimes months ahead.

You have to talk to your professors about the course and the accommodations you might need. You have to get book lists in the summer so you can order your taped texts. People aren't always available when you want to see them. Systems don't always work. Once the audiotape library mixed up the return address with my address and sent my text books to themselves instead of me. As hard as you try, sometimes it doesn't work out and you need a backup plan. I'm still not organized, but I have definitely developed a rough idea of time management.

The thing that helped me with the time pressure was taking a reduced course load. Having three courses instead of five was a big relief, when I was trying to figure out how to study and how the systems worked to get accommodations. Sometimes even then there weren't enough hours in the day to make all those extra arrangements. Over time I got better at handling all the details. Everything and everyone became more familiar. I developed routines. I knew how long things took and when it was time to start making arrangements. I got used to the little snafus that always crop up. I didn't like it, but I got used to it. At least there was a system and I saw the potential. The system got better. By my graduating year, there were enough hours in the day and I took a full five courses like everyone else.

"Your weaknesses and limitations cease to be weaknesses and limitations when you admit them and see them for what they are." I found this quotation in one of my brother's books and I think that translates to almost every aspect of life. I think this is what happened when I started managing my time and my learning style, and getting accommodation. It took me a while to decide to adopt that philosophy. In high school I had this brilliant plan. I'll hide in the bathroom, and this will all sort itself out in a wacky and unpredictable way. It's not my problem anyway. It's their job.

That was my philosophy when I first came to university as well. It will all get sorted out in the wash. But it didn't and I had to switch to the totally opposite attitude. Things are not going to fall into your lap. You have to figure it out for yourself and you have to do it yourself. That's when I started going to professors and talking about my learning style, and planning for the taped texts and taped lectures. After I had done that it wasn't so hard to ask for an exam using the dictaphone. The professors knew I was working hard and that I was interested in the courses. I worked out a deal with the library to keep the specialized four-track tape recorder you needed for books on tape in the music room. I could use it in the library when I was on campus and other students could use it too. Things started happening. My anger dissipated. My marks started improving. It didn't just happen all of a sudden. I didn't just wake up one day and say, "Okay, I've got this all straightened out." It was a gradual thing. It evolved and instead of feeling that I was on the outside of a crystal ball looking in, I felt I had made it inside.

The Social Whirl

After my first assessment at university, I was given a pamphlet about learning disabilities and it pretty much spelled out everything about my life. You are good at this and better at that. When you read something, it doesn't seem to sink in. If something is explained to you, you can understand it. Instructions don't always seem clear. Then there was this part about social skills. How was it worded? People with learning disabilities have a tendency to have low social skills. When someone makes a joke they may not get it, or they may think the joke is on them. They often misinterpret what someone says. That was really a lot like the way I was.

Left on my own, essentially what I did was live in the movies. All of my quotes are from movies, not books. One of the great quotes that meant a lot to me was, "The world was like a crystal ball and I was essentially staring in on it." That's how I felt. I was not in the crystal ball. I was outside of it. I was never directly involved. That's how I really saw school and even university at first. I didn't take the initiative. I never did. I don't know if it was just shyness or, as the pamphlet explained, that I didn't understand. I think it was more that I just didn't understand the social world.

After a while, I began to understand that there were things going on that I just wasn't getting. Two or three days later I would realize that something had happened. What did I do to tick that fellow off? Did that girl make a joke at my expense? Was she just being polite? The majority of this stuff just passes me by, so I tend to remain quiet.

I didn't make friends. People made friends with me. I was just an innocent bystander. One of the people who made friends with me was Rory. He was my ambassador to the social world and my translator or interpreter. I was always Rory's friend or Buddy's brother. I was always the guy in the back seat. I never sat in the front. I never stood out and I never made a spectacle of myself. Some people, even some of my relatives, didn't realize there was a fifth child in my family. I was the guy who never introduced himself. If they didn't talk to me, I didn't talk to them.

When everybody else was into Michael Jackson, I was listening to Led Zeppelin and Jimi Hendrix thanks to my brothers' records.

None of the other kids could believe it at the start, but by the time we were in grade twelve, I was the shining light of our music experience. Everyone wanted to listen to Led Zeppelin then. They had caught up. That was one of the few times I was ahead of everybody else. Rory would say to his friends, "Bob's got that tape." All of a sudden people knew who I was. People would sit down beside me and I had no idea who they were. I thought that they were friends of Rory's, not mine. I couldn't believe that they wanted to hang around with me. Finally they asked Rory why I never introduced myself or talked to them? He passed along the message and then I got it. They wanted to be my friends. That's how I met a lot of the people that are my friends today. These are the same guys who get on my case because I never go out and I never have a girlfriend.

One of the only girls who ever really talked to me was Jean. Now she is a very good friend of mine. At first I thought she was just talking to me because I was a really good friend to her boyfriend. Eventually it became clear to me that she was talking to me because she was interested in what I had to say. Every time I would see her at the bar or somewhere out, I would ask, "Do you mind if I sit down?" Finally she said, "Bob, just sit down. If you ask me that one more time, I'm going to break your nose. How many years do I have to know you before you can just sit with me?" It was just a complete shock to me that she was interested in my companionship. We were friends. WOW! A girl wants to hear what I have to say! She wants to sit and talk to me. I went through university with Jean and she's a great friend. I know that now and I know that I can rely on her. She would explain things to me about social situations. She was my translator and my interpreter.

During these years I rarely went to any of the parties. When I did go, I just kind of hung out in the background. It was the same at bars. People would ask me, "Bob, why don't you go to the bars?" I said, "All I ever do is drink my beer, stare at the floor, and I don't talk to anybody. I can do that at home." They said, "Bob, that's not the point!" I said, "Well, it is to me." In our graduating year, Jean decided it was time to change all that. She took me out, introduced me to people and started me talking to them. She was essentially like an older sister. She would show me what to do, or tell me how to do it.

One of the worst incidents happened a few summers ago. I was in one of the bars in town. There was this girl, whose friend sat beside me in computer science, and she was staring at me. I thought, "Okay, she has recognized me or something." I was sitting with two other fellows and we were talking. I would look over at her every once in a while and she was staring at me, or at least in our direction. I thought, "Obviously she knows the other people." This went on for a while and I thought, "What is going on here?" Finally, I just happened to be walking by that way, and she said, "Hi! How are you doing?" She started asking me all of this stuff, so I said, "Well, I'll see you later." I just couldn't think of anything to say to her. I went away thinking, "She must have me mixed up with someone else." Later I told this story to Jean, and she just started roaring and laughing. She told me the girl was flirting with me. I tried to deny it, but she was convinced. It completely passed me by. Unless you call up and say, "Hi! I like you," it's over my head. I don't notice it one bit, which makes me question how many opportunities I have missed to meet people.

I am more comfortable in smaller groups with people I know well enough to talk to. I went to a dinner for my seminar group at a professor's house. I had never had dinner or a beer, or anything with these people before. A lot of these people had been in classes with me and one girl lives within rock throwing distance of my house. Her father was one of my teachers and we had friends in common, but I had never spoken to her before the seminar. In a small town, where everybody seems to know everybody and things are intertwined, I'm a little paranoid about saying and doing the right thing and hanging around with the right people. I was doubtful that I would ever see many of these people again. That makes it easier for me. In that situation, I'm just the fellow to bring up interesting points and beer makes me extremely talkative. If that dinner had been in September, I wouldn't have said a word, or I probably wouldn't have shown up. It was actually a nice, down to earth occasion for me. From what they tell me, it was quite mellow for the other students sitting around the table and telling stories. It was not like the foolishness they get involved in when they are socializing. For them it was sitting around having a conversation. For me it was a big deal, "I'm socializing. Oh, my God! I'm actually doing something."

I'm not sure how that party appears to me now. I'm not sure how they interpreted me at that party. With Rory or Jean there, I could have asked how I did. They would give me an evaluation or a translation of the situation, and tell me what I should or shouldn't have done. Without that, I'm left wondering. Did they think I was a clown? Were they interested in my viewpoints? Did they just let me speak to be done with it? They laughed when they were supposed to. Were they laughing at me, or at what I said? That's a constant factor in anything I do.

In academics I've learned how to work with people. I've learned how to introduce myself and how to get things done. Sometimes I needed readers for an article or a paper. I had to find people who knew the material better than I did and talk to them about my courses. I figured out that I had things to offer. I could lend my finished notes, help people in the library, or add my view to a discussion. We came to realize each other's strengths and weaknesses. People would come to me with a question and I could go to them. It didn't feel like I was using them. It was more kind of a play off one another, an exchange. I haven't transferred that to social things. It seems too dangerous!

Looking Back

Succeeding at university took a lot of effort and a lot of time, but in many ways it was a lot easier than surviving high school. Let me take you back there.

If I read it doesn't sink in. I don't understand the print until it is told to me. In classes in junior high, I heard the material and I saw things done. It was nice and straightforward. Yet when I went home to study, there was something missing and I didn't understand why. When it came to exams, I would get really angry. I would be trying to study and I would get really frustrated at not being able to do something. Why was I so angry? It was because I couldn't read, but I couldn't really explain why I couldn't read, or what I didn't get out of it. The teacher would ask, "Did you read the material?" "Yes." "What did it say?" All I could answer was, "I don't know!" I would get angry at myself and the teacher would get angry at me for appearing to be slacking off. It would seem obvious to the teacher that I hadn't read the whole thing, I was just saying I had. It seemed obvious to me that I was in an impossible situation.

My strategy was not to draw attention to myself or let people know that I didn't know something. I didn't want to stand out. I was happy in the shadows. I just fit in, but only to a point. I was never in one of the cliques or groups. I didn't dress a certain way to fit in, nothing like that. My motto was, "Don't draw attention to yourself. Don't make mistakes." Otherwise people would then begin to notice and question things. Why was I going to see the teacher on Friday afternoon when everybody under the age of eighteen doesn't want to be within a quarter of a mile of the school? That's when I would take my problems to the teacher. I didn't want to do that in the classroom in front of everyone. I would not. If I didn't know something in class, I would just make a joke of it.

In high school I didn't have any kind of goal or direction. I didn't hate school and I didn't love it. It was just something to do. I would have a boring summer and I'd be eager to get back to school. Then I'd get back, and I couldn't understand what I was reading, and I couldn't understand how I was supposed to be doing things. So one way or another, I just did school. Sometimes I couldn't really care less. At times I just felt angry. I wasn't really angry at anybody else or at myself. I was just angry. I'm not sure if it was because of my learning problem or because I'm just a cranky person. I come from a whole family of cynics. People would ask me why I was so cranky and I would tell them I gave up my sunny disposition for Lent, so leave me alone. In my binder I have written the W.C. Fields quote, "Start every day off with a smile and get the damn thing over with."

Looking back now, it's hard to know just how I was affected by the timing of my assessment and the official diagnosis of my learning disability. I was definitely angry that I had slipped through in my quiet way. I'm not sure who I was angry at. It's always easier to blame someone else rather than yourself. Blame the teachers. For a while I never blamed myself, but why didn't I put up my hand and say, "I don't understand this and I don't know why I don't"? I always just waited for them to find the problem. If they didn't point out the problem, then there was no problem. I'm not sure now who to be angrier with, myself or the teachers. My position was, "It's their job. They should know how to do this stuff." They didn't know and I wasn't able to explain what was going on in my head.

I still feel that sense of frustration at not being able to explain what's going on in my head. When people ask, or I have to explain my situation, I tell them, "I have a learning problem, and it's easier to tell you I'm dyslexic than to try to explain this to you in detail. It would take a year or two." People usually think they know what it means to be dyslexic. They feel it's something they can understand.

Sometimes I think that finding out about my learning disability in university has led me to be a little more independent. I see the system for what it really is and for how it works. I'm not dependent on it. I know that I can function without special assistance. I can see the limitations of my learning style, and of the accommodations and testing system. I know what I am able to accomplish on my own. Before I had any assessments, I thought I was average, nothing spectacular, but now I see that I was being held back. Without these resources and accommodations, I am limited, but I can exist outside the special testing arrangements and the taped texts. I know that I can because I've done it, just not with the same degree of success. I can't excel, but I can manage. I think this makes the ground less shaky for me. I think it also gives me confidence about what comes after university. It's a benefit to know that I can take a job even if they don't offer any special services. If they had special accommodations I would probably do a better job, but I could work without them.

As for the label of learning disabled, I'm not sure how it would have affected me earlier on. I think I would have acted the way I acted, and done what I did, but I think I would have understood my situation better. I think that as things have unfolded, I've become more relaxed and comfortable as I've become more effective at school. If I had been diagnosed in grade two or grade six, I think I would have had this nagging feeling that people were always saying I was special and treating me as special. I hate that term. I think it would have driven me nuts. I think I would have had a lower self-esteem than I do now. As it is, I had to sit across from a department head as she explained to another professor that she had a student with her who was "mentally challenged". The way she went on, it was like someone explaining in front of their dog that they were taking him to the V-E-T! I just sat there and laughed. It seemed so ridiculous to me, but I don't think she understood what I was laughing about. If I had my preference, I think I would probably have things the same way, because I think I might have been worse off from being labelled as special early on. To be labelled as special strikes me as pity, not acceptance.

Last year, I had to get a formal assessment done by a registered psychologist in order to qualify for a government grant to buy a computer of my own. This felt like a big deal to me. By this time, I had completed my degree and I was back at university taking a year of political science courses. I had always paid my own way at university. I had never taken a student loan. I had as little to do with the government and their forms as possible. Then I heard about this program for technological support. I knew how much different my life would be if I had my own computer, so I decided to try to qualify as a person with a disability.

I was really apprehensive. It was the thing about society believing you. I needed documented proof of everything. I had to prove to them, when it was obvious to me, that I had a learning problem. I got very nervous. Maybe I am just lazy? Maybe the tests at university were the one deviation from the truth? Maybe I don't have a learning problem? Maybe it's a lie? Maybe the past four years were just an elaboration of that single lie? Then everything else - the taped texts, the taped lectures, the oral exams, the dictaphone - was just to prove that this lie was real. Sometimes when you're explaining to professors, they are really cooperative and things fall right into place in the course. They just accept you and your situation and try to help. It makes things so easy that I feel like it must be a lie. I guess you could say I was paranoid, but in the days before my assessment, it really felt like it might all have been some kind of a farce. I was afraid I would be humiliated in front of my peers. I would be caught with all that special treatment and I didn't have a problem.

Fortunately, I was proven wrong. I do have a learning disability. Hooray! In a sense I felt vindicated. I was able to prove to these bureaucrats that I did have a learning disability. Here is my proof. Here is my documentation. The first time I had an assessment, I realized I was actually different from everybody else and it was not a very pleasant experience. Over the years I came to accept this fact. I'm a little slower in some areas and a little stronger in others. I can work around it. After the second assessment came around, I thought, "Okay! I have proven myself to everybody else. Rejoice! It's about time this disability started paying its own way."

Success

I consider myself a success at university because I graduated. I made it through. I know what I'm doing and I am capable of going out into the real world that everyone used to talk about. If I had known at the start of university all of the things that would be involved, and all of the things I would wind up doing, I would have said, "I'm out of here! I'd rather panhandle in front of the bank." But that's life and you learn to deal with it.

I don't know how to say this without sounding pompous, but I consider myself very successful. You see, in some respects I may be more successful than other people who graduate, because it wasn't a level playing field for me. I caught up and I got through. Some people I passed along the way and some people are still ahead of me, but essentially I held my ground and gained some too. I was happy to be on the Dean's list, but I didn't expect it. I didn't care so much about marks. Not to sound pompous again, but I know people who get eighties and I know the material better than they do, but I didn't get eighties. My goal was to pass in order to be able to continue learning.

What did I learn at university? I learned that the system does not work on its own. You have to make it work for you. I learned that you won't get anything done unless you ask somebody. I found that you learn more from your mistakes than you ever will from your accomplishments. (Why am I speaking as though I'm writing greeting cards?)

It wasn't so much what I learned in classes, but the peripheral issues. I learned how to budget time, plan ahead, set deadlines for myself and not just do things ad hoc or put them off. I know things aren't going to just get done on their own. I know they're not just going to fall into my lap. I learned that I was a lot more capable than I gave myself credit for. An eight-page paper? It almost seems simplistic now. I also learned how to work with people. You can tie all those things into getting a job. In a job interview, I'm sure they will be asking me about what I can and cannot do. I'll be very honest. I know what I can do, and now I know that I can ask and there will be someone who can show me, or I can figure out some way of getting most things done.

I came back to the university after I graduated and gave a talk to some high school students with learning disabilities. It was a good feeling. I felt I was in the loop and I had come full circle. I was part of things. It wasn't just me on the outside of the crystal ball looking in. I felt that it could happen for them too. In choosing a university I told them to look for three things: a system for special accommodations (you don't need a huge staff, but there should be a system); access to tutors; and someone who knows what's going on and sees things from your perspective. It's always nice to have somebody in your corner who can help you plan and argue your case.

Sometimes I'm surprised I stuck it out at university. In my family you don't expect things to be easy. If it's too easy, it must be wrong. Maybe that helped me stay with it, that and my conservative nature. There are no burnt out light bulbs in my family. All five of us picked the kind of education we wanted and did it. No pressure. I picked the road I wanted and I stayed on it.

THE VIEW FROM OUTSIDE

When I first saw Bob, he looked like a typical student in his jeans and jean jacket. He seemed quiet, perhaps shy, but certainly hesitant and unconvinced that he should be talking to me. Even though Bob had initiated the meeting with me through his English professor, he seemed to be having second thoughts. Once we began talking about his reading and learning strategies, many of the typical features of a student with a learning disability began to emerge.

What also began to appear was a thoughtful young man who was determined, willing to work and eager to learn. Intuitively, Bob had come up with some good coping strategies and had managed to graduate from high school with a 70 per cent average. He was using books on tape from the local library for his pleasure reading and he loved watching films. He had set up a plan following high school that allowed him to upgrade his math skills and try some university courses in preparation for a science program in engineering. He thought he could use his ability and experience in carpentry to advantage in engineering, while minimizing the amount of essay writing and the kind of reading done in arts courses. He had talked his way into a graphics course which was not generally allowed for students outside of engineering. He had decided that computer science and English would be useful to him. I think he also sensed that the English course might give him a chance to sort out his reading and writing problems. He had even managed to get to my office before his first term at university was over. I saw a young man with a lot going for him, who was floundering in his struggle to cope with university work.

Bob already had the habit of taking his strengths and weaknesses into account and trying to find ways around the obstacles he encountered. Bob's reasoning through these problems seemed excellent to me, given the amount of information he had. I was impressed with the amount of effort he was willing to expend. Clearly Bob needed some more information about how he learned, and some discussion about different options he could use to maximize his strengths and accommodate his weaknesses.

Over the Christmas break Bob and I completed some formal testing. Here is how I summarized the results:

> *Bob is currently in the bright normal range of intellectual functioning. His subtest scores show scatter consistent with his difficulties in reading and writing skills. He has significant strength in both verbal and spatial abstract reasoning. He appears to be well informed and thoughtful about the world around him. The testing suggests that he would be a good candidate for university if it were not for his reading and writing deficits. The Davis Reading Test indicates severe difficulties in reading*

speed and comprehension of college level material.

This initial assessment reveals a pattern consistent with the diagnosis of learning disability. It would be useful to pursue further testing to understand more clearly the processing difficulties Bob is experiencing. Tests of verbal and auditory memory may provide significant information. Bob is eager to understand and remediate his reading and writing skills.

Further assessment was not immediately available. Finding a registered psychologist who did evaluations for adults and finding the money to pay for it was only a part of the problem. Bob was not sure what he wanted to do about pursuing the idea of being learning disabled. Bob and I just continued to talk about his current learning situation, as well as the latest movies. We discussed strategies that might make him a more effective learner at university. We discussed trade school. Our contact was intermittent. Bob would get his appointment times mixed up. He might come early, or he might come late. Sometimes he came on the wrong day. Gradually he began to call ahead to check, or drop in after to apologize. When he did get in for an appointment, he sat across from me looking like he was being tortured. It was impossible for him to stay more than twenty minutes.

At this point Bob seemed to be sorting through the new information he had and he was trying various experiments to deal with his problems with print. We had all sorts of logistical and bureaucratic problems to occupy us like finding tape recorders, notetakers, tutors, text books on tape, or readers. We would discuss what worked and what did not. Bob would find new things to try. He might not have looked like he was enjoying himself, but he certainly was not giving up.

Bob completed his first year at university as a part-time student, with 60 per cent in English, 59 per cent in graphics and a failing grade in computer programming. His high school mathematics courses had gone very well. He decided to return to university full time in the fall to try a combination of science and arts courses. Since he had still not ruled out engineering, he took calculus and physics, two of the required courses for that program. He carried on with a higher-level English course, and decided to try the social sciences with psychology and sociology. Bob continued experimenting with learning strategies, although he did not use any special exam provisions. He was willing to change the things he could do on his own, but he did not want to talk to professors about his learning style, or ask for "special" treatment from them.

Things did not run smoothly. After Christmas, Bob withdrew from physics in an attempt to lighten his work load and save his academic average. He did not want to give up on calculus although it was not going well either. He was struggling academically on all fronts. Some of his adjustments were starting to pay off, but not in time to make much impact on his final grades. Bob finished the year with a dramatic 20 per cent in calculus and squeaked out a pass in his other courses with a high of 58 per cent in modern English literature. After making an appeal to the dean of arts, he was placed on academic probation and given a chance to continue in the arts program.

This was a critical summer for Bob. He had to give up on engineering as a career goal and studying science as a solution to his learning barriers. He started using some accommodation strategies, but it was not easy. He had to do a lot more planning and organization if that was going to work well. Somewhere in there, he checked out trade school again and got some more formal learning evaluations done. I was getting ready to go on leave for the upcoming academic year. We talked about all of the problems involved in setting up the things he needed to accommodate his learning style. I wrote a letter to support his appeal to continue in the Arts program. I listened to the list of grievances he had about failures in the system. I knew that they were legitimate complaints and that they were unlikely to disappear entirely. We talked about planning to take the flaws into account. He listened to me tell him to take control and make the necessary things happen. When I went on my leave, I did not know whether Bob would stay at university or not.

On my return a year later, I was delighted to find Bob at our Centre lining up taped texts for his next four courses. It was well before the start of term and he had already interviewed most of his professors. He was no longer on academic probation. He had a comfortable 63 per cent average for his last three courses and was now an English major. He had carefully selected his courses to capitalize on his learning strengths, and the availability of tutorial and notetaking support from his friends. He had even managed to get a spot in the highly subscribed film course. As a career option, he was considering work with young offenders when he graduated. By the end of that year, Bob's name was on the dean's list for academic achievement.

The year was not without the usual frustrations, but Bob worked very hard. He was getting better at showing what he had learned, and we were getting a better system for arranging taped texts and exam accommodations. We were all learning. Bob and I continued to review the problems of being a special student, usually by discussing a movie. We had a lot of running jokes from the film *What About Bob?,* where the patient relentlessly pursues the psychiatrist until finally the roles are reversed. Bob still felt uncomfortable with his status and very uncomfortable about getting help. He was particularly hesitant about using a style of testing different from his classmates. It almost seemed his reservations were because it had been so effective in changing his academic prospects.

In his graduating year, Bob took a full course load. He posted a 68 per cent average and developed an interest in political science. I think he might have maintained his status on the Dean's List if he had taken a reduced course load, but he wanted to test his strength and see what he could do with five courses like everyone else. He visited me for check-in sessions and worked with a specialized tutor on his writing skills. The rest seemed to be business as usual. Things went more smoothly and Bob was an excellent role model for the incoming students. His low key, cynical style went over very well with them. He also gave us a hand with a project to upgrade the library facilities for students with disabilities. He still barely endured our social functions, but he came back after his graduation to give a presentation to high school students with learning disabilities. He was great! In a structured situation where he understood his role he could shine.

After looking at the employment opportunities, Bob decided to return for further studies in political science and to take another try at a computer course. He also wanted to get a formal assessment so that he could qualify for a technology grant from the provincial government. I think he was not ready to move on yet. He wanted some more chances at academic success, and the opportunity to try a fourth-year seminar course where he could prepare and present a research paper.

I have always been impressed by Bob's intellectual curiosity. In spite of his problems with print, he is very much suited to an academic life. He likes to learn, and will expend a tremendous amount of energy to get access to ideas and new information. To pay for his tuition, Bob worked in the woods planting trees or cutting pulp. He made his pocket money doing painting and maintenance work. He refused to go into debt to attend classes, but he always seemed to be able to come up with a sensible plan that allowed him to continue to learn.

I think Bob had a very productive and enjoyable final year at university, in his own low key way. He was a valuable asset to our program once again. He was an effective mentor to the younger students. He was immensely helpful with the logistics of securing taped texts and he helped us train volunteer readers. He also did volunteer work for the county's Citizens Coalition for Persons with Disabilities. He participated in our employment seminars and was part of a panel presentation on learning disabilities at a faculty education session. He secured some part-time work at the library that expanded his job experiences. He earned a satisfying 76 per cent in his seminar course. He was officially diagnosed as a student with a learning disability and managed to sort his way through the paper work of getting his grant. He was able to buy a computer complete with the adaptive technology he needs for dealing with print. When Bob graduated the previous year, he had been sick "with the plague" for all of the celebrations and claimed that he had only barely managed to walk across the stage for his degree. This time he went to the parties. He was finally beginning to add social successes to his academic ones. He picked the road he wanted and he has come miles.

For most of his school life Bob escaped notice. His account describes vividly the distance his learning style put between him and the rest of his world. He felt "trapped outside the crystal ball". Bob is bright, analytical and a keen observer. However, to most of his teachers he appeared lazy and unmotivated. Nothing could have been further from the truth. To deal with a situation that left him feeling confused and angry, he used all kinds of creative approaches. He managed to find enough connections to survive and carve out a quirky, cynical persona that let him pass through situations without having to display the difficulties that he was experiencing. In a sense he was too successful at this. It was not until his failures at university that he was forced into changing his policy of passive participation. It was there that he also found people who were willing to see his strengths and help him find ways of expressing them.

At university, it was necessary for Bob to come out of hiding and take action in a new way in order to stay on. It was not easy for him to change his style and it was not easy for me to understand enough about what was going on beneath that crusty exterior to be helpful. Many times I'm sure I was not very helpful, but he knew that I was trying. Luckily, Bob was not accustomed to progress being quick or easy. He was tremendously determined to work things out once he had found a new perspective with some possibilities for success. He changed his life dramatically, one step at a time. He has grown into a life that suits him even though it seemed unlikely, especially to him. I hope that those trapped and lonely years that Bob spent will give you renewed interest in reaching out to the quiet resisters around you.

5
BOB MACDONALD
World of Work

I met with Bob on a sunny autumn day in the city in Western Canada that is his home. He seemed unchanged even though he was now in his forties. He still favoured shirts and jeans like the ones he has always worn. His humorous cynical style remained too. He gave me a great tour of the sights of his new city and was clearly enthusiastic about some of the activities and entertainments on offer. He continues to be interested in history and politics and filled me in on some of the local issues and the changes and progress that were underway. He appeared settled and content in his job as a university librarian. At university he had learned to use and enjoy libraries and he began to see them as an environment where he could make a career for himself. There were many twists and turns before he reached his goal but he picked the road he wanted and persisted. Seeing him today made me feel that it was a very good choice. Here is how it worked out.

Finding a Career

When I finished high school I wanted to become an engineer. That took me to university. There I realized engineering was just not going to work for me. After a few attempts at other courses, I realized I really liked English and Political Science. I had avoided that stuff because of the reading but once I figured out how to manage the reading and the notes, I could enjoy those subjects and do pretty well. This is when I discovered the library. It was my kind of place. I thought maybe I could work there. After I graduated, I got a grant and a placement at my university library to see how I would fit. I tried all the different jobs over the course of the year. I got pretty positive feedback but there were no vacancies.

Next I went to community college and did a library technician course. I thought it might improve my chances of getting a job. The course had practicum placements and I got to see and work in different kinds of libraries. I got good references and I was offered a job from there at a government staff training centre. It meant moving but I wanted the work. Surprisingly, I enjoyed the change of environment. It was different from working at my university in my hometown. I had a free hand in organizing their collection and they really liked what I did. People about my age came and worked on short courses involving international development and peace keeping. The faces were always changing. I made interesting friends. I got to travel with them as part of the job.

I know I didn't say anything about my learning disability in my interview for that job. I never really did identify myself. This was my first serious job as a professional librarian. It was kind of a pressure job and I didn't declare because I wanted to prove my merits to myself and to them. In case I screwed something up, I didn't want to make it sound like I had a ready-made excuse as to why I was doing a terrible job. As it turned out I never had to disclose. My disability wasn't an issue. I really enjoyed working there and things went well. The only reason I left was that they closed the place down. The job ended but I got the sense that I had found a career that I could be good at. I had the references and the experience to prove it.

Jobs turned out to be pretty scarce. I did this and that to pay the bills and kept looking. It seemed that there were few library jobs around and the ones I wanted required a degree in library science. I saved up and went to do a master's degree in library science at a university in Ontario. I researched the program for students with disabilities and got myself enrolled before I left home. This was a big difference from the way I wandered into university the first time. It worked way better, even though I went there without knowing anyone. The academic program was intense but I managed. I got through all the hurdles and became a professional librarian. It helped that I already knew a lot about libraries and library jobs. Another thing was that I made one really good friend there. She was usually my partner in assignments. We worked well together. She went back out West and I went home to the East. We were both hoping we could get jobs in the same area but it didn't happen.

Now that I was a full-fledged librarian with a master's degree, it seemed that everybody in Nova Scotia could only afford a technician and I was over qualified. I did all kinds of jobs that I was overqualified for just to support myself. I worked in the woods, proctored exams, pumped gas and shelved books as a casual worker. In the meantime, I kept applying for jobs as a librarian. My goal was to work in a university library.

Getting the Job

What really started things moving in the right direction for my job search was a call from my brother in Calgary. He called me up and said "You have a master's degree and you're pumping gas in Nova Scotia for eight dollars and ten cents an hour. Out here there's a fast-food chain that will pay you sixteen bucks an hour. Besides I need someone to house sit. I think you should get out here." I said okay.

I came out West and to my surprise I saw all these job ads. One of the good things about libraries is that they like to share all of their information including the job postings. I went to a couple of career servers and I applied for library jobs. There was a posting for a position at a university library. Within a month of arriving I was hired part-time at the university. Eventually my position became full-time. Until that happened, I found another part-time job at a public library. I didn't care for it but it paid some bills. Suddenly people would hire me.

I couldn't really believe this was happening. Before I moved out West, I couldn't get a librarian job. I had good references. I had other librarians as mentors. They helped me with my resume and practice interviews and I still got nothing. I would get to know people and show them what I could do so they would give me a chance and even then there often didn't seem to be money to hire me. I suppose it was a bit like that here with moving from part-time to full-time positions but I did get both of those part-time jobs straight from an ad. It wasn't my usual experience. It seems I just had to be in the right place to get the work I wanted. My learning disability didn't seem to be an issue.

Getting a Good Fit

When it comes to a job interview, there will usually be something along the lines of name your strengths and weaknesses and that's usually where I identify my learning disability. I say "I'm a production person. I get things started but the niggly little details aren't my strongest suit. Having a learning disability, I realize that my strength is not in the details and following procedures in a set way. I may have to make a few adjustments but I am good at delivering the product." That's typically how I would handle an interview situation. My learning disability is identified and usually that is the only time it's discussed.

I've had all kinds of jobs. In some I have identified myself as a person with a disability and in some I haven't. I've had all kinds of jobs. For some places I can't actually remember what I did. Over time it doesn't seem that important. At my current position in the university library I have basically mentioned my learning disability in the interview and then casually in conversation so people I work with know. It makes things more comfortable. I think now people are much more understanding and sympathetic to other people who need something different.

I know I need a job where you don't have to produce written reports on a regular basis. The submission of written reports or anything beyond verbal discussions isn't really something that I've had to deal with a lot in my jobs. I don't know if that's where I purposely put myself or if it is just happenstance but usually the jobs I've had don't require much report writing.

I am very satisfied with the job I have now. I have a position where all I do is answer questions and train students. I have lots of experience with clarifying questions, checking all of the options and keeping things simple. It's how I managed to get my degrees. As a librarian I help find books and articles. I find them. I don't have to read them so my print problems are minimal. Being able to find things seems to me to be an obvious part of a librarian's job. But apparently I'm very good at it and not everybody is. I never really thought it was all that magical.

In some jobs you don't have that same magic. There was this job in a public library that I took when I first came out West. As it turned out I happened to despise it. Unlike my current job, I was called a librarian but the job was really all about crowd control and monitoring the use of the computers. There were a lot of people around with no place to go and they used this library for a hang out. I always seemed to be the one who had to check on what was really going on in the corners or in the washrooms. That could be unpleasant. So I was glad when I was able to walk away from that one.

Now a lot of my job is explaining to people how the data bases work. I guess in a way it is teaching. I do this with the library users and with the student staff. For example, someone comes to the desk and they tell me they are doing a paper on exercise and autism. I'll tell them where they can look if they want to work on this topic. I don't actually do the work for them. I show them how it's done. I know how important it is to be able to work independently. Usually I will explain everything by using a search for Marco Polo. The funny thing is some people get that joke and some people don't. Saying that I'm looking for Marco Polo amuses me anyhow. When I'm training the student staff I set up themes for the week or contests for little known facts or obscure resources. It adds some entertainment for all of us and makes a good team. I enjoy working with the students.

With my current job there has only been one time that my learning disability was an issue and the problem was resolved in a very short time. I was transferred to the Cancer Center to work for the medical sciences side of the library. I guess it was a bit of a promotion but I was completely out of my realm. There, everything needed to have all of the t's crossed and the i's dotted. They had a vocabulary I knew nothing about. Do you realize that cancer is actually called neoblast? I never did. I had never even heard the term before and there were lots more like that. The kind of language and that level of detail didn't really suit me. It was like trying to learn a whole new way of seeing. It was agreed after about two months that I was doing a terrible job so I moved back to the main university library. There was no fuss at all.

The reason I had to leave the Cancer Center Library was that I couldn't catch on to the language and the details of how things are organized and found. My brain doesn't work that way. In the main library, I enjoy hearing about and thinking about all the projects that people are trying to tackle. Here I'll find all the stuff people need and sometimes I can point out other sources they hadn't thought about using. I can't explain to you exactly how I do it but it seems straightforward to me.

Managing a Learning Disability

You can learn how to manage in all kinds of ways. Through trial and error I learned how to manage on my own at high school. Once I got to university I found out more about how I learned. I found a whole new set of things to try and people to talk to about learning disabilities. There were new skills and technology on offer. I realized that things won't just fall into your lap but you can ask someone and probably figure out ways of getting most things done. When I started taking control and making changes things started happening. My marks started improving. I didn't feel angry all the time. I had better things to do. I developed routines and things started to go more smoothly. It didn't happen in a day. It was a gradual thing. When I graduated from university on the dean's list it made me feel that I knew what I was doing. I had learned that I could succeed and I was ready to take my chances out there in the real world that everyone talks about. I did that and mostly it has all worked out.

Not too long ago I was thinking about one of the lessons I learned from books. I read a historian's account of the building of the

Brooklyn Bridge and the Panama Canal. This fellow, by the name of David Laughlin I think, wrote in a style that was part history channel, part discovery channel and a lot of science too. Anyway, it's a long story, but the part that I want to mention was that they planned to spend almost three years just doing infrastructure before they started building the Canal. One of the chief engineers was asked "Why did it take three years?" He said it was because of something his arithmetic teacher taught him. "If you get a problem and it takes ten minutes to solve it, it takes the first seven minutes just to figure out how you are going to do it. You don't just start digging."

I think this story caught my attention because I never did like just to dive right in. At first, when I started out doing assignments I used to dive right in and muck about and usually make a bloody mess before I finally got things straightened out. Now I plan the steps. I sit back and figure out how I'm actually going to do a project. Maybe it looks like I'm procrastinating and I probably am doing some of that too. I think about what the project is going to look like and then I start doing the process. In a way that's what I try to show people who come to the reference desk.

I started to see this strategy work at university and it got me through my graduate program. Now it has carried over into my job. By Tuesday I've got to make a finding guide for one of the software programs that we use for searching out source materials. I was given the task last Thursday. I haven't even touched it yet but I am thinking about it. What am I going to do? What's it going to look like? What information do I want? I'd say that even though I haven't done anything that anyone could see, I've already figured it out.

This kind of strategy isn't specifically for someone with a learning disability. Some people, when they write a paper, like to use cue cards or draw an idea map or dictate from an outline. The process I've described isn't so much the way I prefer to do projects but more the way I should do them because I get a better mark or a better result that way. It's not even the way I'm more comfortable and it doesn't mean it's the best way for everyone. I figure people should use what works best for them.

At work I have meetings with my supervisor on a regular basis to give her my reports orally and to keep in touch. I do still have trouble with spelling and handwriting. For me *a, e, i, o and u* are still optional letters and I think they always will be. I'm not too worried. It's a little bit that I have had more practice getting into print so I am better at it. The other thing is that I write for myself. I don't care if anyone else can read what I write down or not. I've pretty much created my own kind of dialect or language in script. If anything has to be submitted in print, I've got to put it on a computer. I usually hand write everything first. If I don't have the time, I do it on the computer in point form.

Suppose I had to write a report. I might submit an opening draft and say here are all my points, here is the direction I'm going. The thing is, this would be the third or fourth draft but I'll do it about eight times anyway. I always want people who are aware of the basics to check out what I am trying to say. I don't want to put all this energy in if what I'm saying is crap and I have misunderstood something fundamental about the task. As long as the points are made and everything is on topic, I will do several drafts more to get it right. Then I read it out loud to get it to sound right. This system takes time and effort but it's what I used at university. I know I can get good results with it. If I used dictation software that might be easier but I have never really tried it. From what I've heard it has improved immensely in the last twenty years. I probably would find it useful, but as I said, I'm so used to working without it that I just go with the way I always do these things. Since I rarely have to do a formal written report it isn't much of a problem.

I think I could easily get any technology I asked for here, along with a supervisor to strategize with me. But I just don't naturally use any of it. Having said that, I don't know for sure. I have never asked. I've learned to do without fancy accommodations so that's what I feel comfortable doing. They gave me an I-pad and I hate the damn thing. That's the way I feel about using a lot of technology. I can recommend programs for others and I even teach students how to use some of them. But I don't use any kind of gadgets personally. I still write everything down the way I always did.

I have asked for some adjustments in my current job and it has worked out well. For example, I would naturally avoid staff meetings if I could. I find staff meetings a lot like lectures. I don't pick up the information very well and the social and political dynamics confuse me even more. Someone needs to be out front to cover the desk while everyone else goes to the meeting so I volunteered. I worked it out with my supervisor to make this part of my routine duties. She fills me in on things that involve my work and things she feels I should know after the meeting. Other staff members don't want me to miss the action so they are usually happy to offer me their analysis of the meeting too. This is what I mean about making adjustments. I don't stress myself out trying to get through the meeting and it seems to give me better working relationships with everyone too.

The Social Whirl

I remember always feeling isolated and kind of off on my own. To this day, I'd much rather go for a walk in the snow by myself than do any number of things with a bunch of people. I'm not sure if that is something in my personality that was always there or just what would have evolved out of my learning situation. There are a few people that I like and who seem to like me. Usually we have some interest in common or some quirky ideas that we share. That's enough for me.

I'm still not much of a risk taker when it comes to social occasions. I have taken risks like moving around the country for work and trying new jobs but that all had to do with necessity. Mostly I believe in sticking a toe in first, to test things out. I'll drag my feet on pretty much anything. When someone arrives in town from my hometown and I haven't seen them in a while, sure, I'll go for a cup of coffee or give them a place to stay. But I'm probably not going to go to the pub or a club or anything like that. Now everyone realizes that when I say, "Sure, I'll show up." I'm not going to show up. I just say that so they will stop bothering me. That way we can all feel good that they asked.

You see I can't stand meeting up with a dozen people in someplace crowded and noisy. I just start crawling the walls. It makes me feel like I'm alone inside the bubble again. I still get that feeling. Now I'm a little more aware of that fact so I don't put myself through those kinds of events. In many cases, I'm just not a very sociable person. I'd like to be, but I'm just not. I'm completely naïve in some situations. It's not the fact that I don't have a social interpreter like in the old days. I've had the opportunity to learn all your social rules and skill sets and I let it go right by. I suppose I still have time to catch up but I really don't feel like doing it. I'm also at a time in my life when I can do more of the things that make me feel good, and I don't have to push myself like that.

What I like to do, a lot of people wouldn't call a social life. I have my few, little happy places where I like to go and that's about it. I am still a big movie fan and there is a repertory cinema that I go to all the time. I've got my favourite restaurants and bars. At one of the bars I go to regularly they call me the librarian. I order a Guinness and a pen and I'll sit there in a crowded bar and I'll do the Sudoku and watch the hockey game. I won't talk to anybody except for a couple of the other regulars. I'll wave at them and ask what's going on but normally I just keep to myself. That's the kind of thing I'm most comfortable with.

I guess it's a bit surprising but I like hosting my student workers when we do what they call our team building activities. I know my role as the designated adult and I'm comfortable with it. I've also made some friends through work and I take road trips for an afternoon or go hiking with them. I've joined an archery group with some of my brother's friends. I'm not very good at it but I find the sport really interesting and I like the company. Where I'm in a structured social situation with a purpose and a time frame it's easier for me to relax. I feel I know what I'm doing and how to participate.

Every year I try to make it back home to see the rest of my family and the old crowd. Even so everyone complains that I don't keep in touch enough. Usually around Halloween, I take vacation time and go to a big city like New York, San Francisco or London. It's my tradition. I'll research the place or I will already have some reason why I want to go there. Sometimes I want to visit friends I have met on previous trips. I always travel alone and I always meet interesting people. I usually have an adventure or two. As a guy who grew up in small town, I love big cities. I have a long list of cities to sample so this should keep me busy for a while.

Looking Back

I was wondering if my thoughts on life had changed since I graduated from university. I looked back at my comments from that time. My ideas about taking control, stepping forward, identifying yourself, getting into the system, all that stuff, still seem pretty much something I would agree with today. Those pieces of advice are actually something I mentioned last night to the student workers I supervise at the library. Essentially the idea is just to get in front of things. Have a go. If you screw up let the right person know. If you've got a problem, always ask a question. Never wait on it. I tell them the same things now that I thought were important then in getting me going in the right direction. It's still something I pay attention to even though I didn't always do things that way myself. With or without a disability those pieces of advice are important things to keep in mind. I use them myself now and it seems to work out.

If I look back at what happened to me in school, I would say there seems to be more understanding of learning disabilities now. It wasn't until I got to university that my learning disability was recognized. I was told in high school that there were no tests in the whole school board system that could figure out my problems. I wasn't failing so the teachers seemed to think my marks were good enough. I had one teacher who was convinced that I had a learning disability and that was it. No one else identified that I might have a learning problem. No one else even looked at how I learned or why I couldn't do better.

I think learning disabilities are much more identified now. I hear that students are being tested at early ages. I like to think that someone like me wouldn't slip through the cracks in the same way as I did. People might know that maybe that boy is not just lazy. They might see that there's more to it than being a slow reader or a poor speller. Maybe that student needs more than a little extra time. I don't know what they do in the elementary school systems these days. I hope there is some sort of program to help. They should make some kinds of adjustments and find a way to teach and grade you. They should do something so you can get credit for what you can do and what you have learned. I'm not sure what would help but I think having people there who do know and understand more is really important.

Now I definitely feel that it would be better to be identified with a learning disability earlier than I was. I don't know that it would have changed me any but I probably would have had a better skill set and picked up the skills I needed earlier. It might have saved me a lot of grief and frustration. Sometimes I think that only finding out about my learning disability in university has led me to be a little more independent. I can see the limitations of the support systems. I know that I can function without special assistance. I may be limited but I can manage. It's a benefit to know that I could probably take a job even if they don't offer any special accommodations. I know what I am able to accomplish on my own and I know that I can do well in the right job.

At the university where I work now, they are aware of learning disabilities. They have a program and a system of supports for the students. In the library, one of our meeting rooms is designated specifically for students with learning disabilities. They can meet there with their counsellors or other students to work on their projects. The students do use the room but not particularly for the equipment. A lot of the new stuff like Dragon Dictate, Beacon Write, Read to Me or PDF readers can all be put on a flash drive and carried around. Mostly you don't need the special technology room any more. You just need a flash drive and a computer which most people have these days. The technology situation has really improved since my day.

In the end, the room in the library is used mainly for meeting with strategists. What these strategists do I'm not exactly sure. I think they work towards teaching students what to focus on, how to organize their assignments, how to write a paper, and some skill sets for studying. I assume it's something along those lines. I hope they do because those are all the kinds of things that I had to figure out at university. That's how I learned what to do when I am given any assignment and those skills have transferred over to my career.

When I left university, I still felt some of that anger and a sense of frustration at not being able to explain what was going on in my head. It wasn't easy. I had to try different things, get more education and move around the country. At the start, my strategy used to be not to draw attention to myself or let people know that I didn't know something. I didn't want to talk about what I couldn't do. I was hiding behind what I could do. I would try to make a joke if I got caught out. I think that is one of the important things that I have changed. I'm much more relaxed about the whole thing now.

In the past, I was used to giving talks about disabilities but I haven't really stuck with doing anything like that where I live now. Before I had steady work here, I used to proctor exams at the disability resource centre, but that's about all the contact I had around my disability. I think if I was asked, I might give a talk but I have not specifically gone out and looked for opportunities. This wasn't by design. I just kind of evolved into a place where having a learning disability wasn't the first thing on my mind. I consider it like having curly hair or being left-handed or being one of those crazy people with a nose ring. It's the situation and it's just part of your growing up. I don't see myself as a person with a learning disability who is a librarian. I see myself as a librarian who lives out West and who's worked here and there. I also have a learning disability so I'm a slow reader and I have to make a few adjustments. I guess that's the way I always saw it.

I do think the stigma has changed for the better. I don't feel that negative stereotype is still there in the same way as it was twenty years ago. I know another guy with a learning disability who like me is kind of surprised at how well he is received. People are interested in what we have to offer as opposed to when we were starting out. Now using the term is almost like saying you have celiac disease or you are a vegan or something like that with dietary restrictions. People are much more aware and sympathetic to other people who need something different. I wouldn't want to push that too far though. Maybe it's partly a function of our age and experience and that we keep learning better coping skills. Having said that, it's still always stressful trying to cope with a new situation but it's easier than it used to be.

Looking Forward

My goal was to be a librarian and work in a university library. Now I do. The job I have is the best. The pay isn't that great but everyone always thinks their pay should be better. I really do like what I do now. It's always changing. I like the challenge of finding good resources for people and showing them how to do the research themselves. In a way my job stays the same but it's always changing. Some days I may get asked the same question three or four times, but not in a row and not by the same person in the same way. You have to learn how to deal with all the situations as they come up and all the issues that confuse people. These are the things that I enjoy teaching to the student assistants I supervise.

This job is one of the few that didn't evolve out of a job placement or a situation where people had known me for a while and knew they wanted to hire someone like me. These people didn't know me at all. That makes me feel more comfortable about what I can do. I like knowing that now I can see a position advertised, compete and get the job. Even though I don't want to leave this job, it makes me feel like getting employment would be less of a struggle if I did.

I'm comfortable living in this big city and I enjoy the people I work with. There are lots of walking trails, events and places to check out. I've gotten to know the area and some of the history of the place. I follow the ways they are working on urban development. My brother is moving back to Nova Scotia but I want to stay on here. I am looking for a new place to live. I have found a neighbourhood I like. It's close enough to my work and it seems like a real community with lots of little shops and restaurants and kind of a counter culture feeling. A little apartment on my own there, not too big to take care of, would suit me just fine.

In the end, I think the main thing for a person with a learning disability is to find out what works for you and go from there. It's important not to worry about your differences but be aware of them and accept what works for you and what doesn't. If you do that, things just carry on to the point where your disability doesn't really exist anymore. It's just something you do. It's your routine and you don't even have to think about it. If there is one thing I want to emphasize it's not to be too worried about being different. The times have changed. It's trendy now to be different. It makes you interesting.

THE VIEW FROM OUTSIDE

Would you predict that a person with a learning disability would find a satisfying career as a university librarian? You would also be surprised that a person who did not have many positive experiences in his first fourteen years of schooling still believed in the power and promise of education. So much so that he earned not one but two university degrees and a college diploma as well. Yet that is what happened. Bob learned how to succeed as a student and developed a range of professional competencies that brought him both career opportunities and job satisfaction. He has found his way through periods of being ignored, misunderstood, angry and frustrated to a place and way of being in the world that he enjoys.

It was a lonely struggle for Bob to find the keys to success in a classroom but his persistence and determination have clearly paid off. He has used to good advantage the lessons he learned about himself through all of those challenges. It is hard not to link his focus on self-reliant strategies with those early years of struggle on his own. Now you can hear how his comfort and confidence have grown. Once he settled on the goal of being a librarian he put himself in learning situations where he could experience first-hand the workings and skills used in different settings and aspects of the profession. He used his time at community college to get further practical training and experience. This opened the way to his first job as a librarian managing a collection on his own. When that road was blocked he decided to improve his credentials. When he went off to university this time, he had an understanding of his learning style and strategies. He registered in advance with the program for students with disabilities. He had a plan and a system. This was a very big change from the way he started his post-secondary studies. It was still difficult, hard work but he made a good working partnership and found his way through.

Although he claims to be risk averse, Bob has moved house and province several times for the sake of his career without being "too worried about it". He regards those changes as a necessary choice and yet another project with some new and interesting challenges. This attitude seems to carry over to his enjoyment of travelling on his own and exploring new places. Interestingly the risk Bob has not taken is the risk of trying new technology. On the surface it seems a change of strategy might help him a great deal with the production of written reports. Instead he chooses the comfort of his proven ways in a job that requires almost no paper work. He doesn't mind putting in the extra time and he is comfortable asking for editorial support. His ideal job allows him the choice.

Bob has adopted a simple straightforward approach to thinking about and explaining his learning disability and perhaps to his life in general. He has found ways of avoiding the pressure of a crowded social life and established a comfortable network of friends and activities. He has been able to manage in a variety of employment situations usually with little or no accommodation from the employer. This is important to him. He places a high value on self-reliance. When a serious problem about his job performance arose after a transfer, Bob was able to sort it out without conflict or bad feelings. The feeling that he can successfully compete for a job on the basis of his skills and credentials and do that job well has given him a fundamental sense of security.

When Bob's library was designated as a safe haven for local people after an extreme weather event, Bob was put in charge of organizing the temporary housing for the homeless. One more time he faced a problem, made a plan and saw it through. It seems clear that Bob's employers recognize and value his skills and he enjoys offering them. Socially, Bob may keep his distance but he is not without connections and friends. Every work day he goes off to university and sits in the middle of a vast store of information and helps people learn how to use it. He found the job he hoped for in an environment where learning and difference is "trendy" and he fits right in.

6
JOHN CARPENTER
University Years

My name is John Carpenter. I graduated from university with a Bachelor's degree in Business Administration, along with two hundred other students. I have a major in accounting. I would describe myself as very intensely focused and task-oriented. I have a million ideas and my mind is always going at one hundred and ten percent. When I am focusing I can forget about everything else, but if I get a distraction, off I go. I completely lose what I'm doing. My train of thought just goes. This can be detrimental, but it didn't stop me from getting my degree.

I have a learning disability and I have attention deficit disorder (ADD) or hyperactivity. The ADD means I really can't stay focused on too much of anything for too long. If somebody walks by outside, I'll look at what's going on outside. I'll admire the sights and take a scenic tour. Then I'll look back at the speaker, the picture on the desk, the chair. I can't focus on one thing for an overly long period of time. I get intense focuses. Then I'll get distracted and lose my thought processes. I'll forget the question. As you can imagine, this doesn't exactly make it easy to be a student.

Apparently, I also have some form of reading problem which I still haven't figured out. My memory is pretty interesting too. Short bits of information go right over my head. I can forget what someone said to me ten seconds ago. I'm terrible at taking lecture notes, but give me twelve hours to process a lecture and I can recite it. My nickname is "Crayola Crayons" because I use crayons to make coloured lecture notes that I can follow. Sometimes I think I have problems with communication. I often wonder if I really got my message across.

I can get frustrated easily, but I am very determined. I can come across as extremely stubborn and argumentative. At some points these can be strengths. It depends on the situation. I don't give up and that's got me through a lot of tough spots. A good argument can get you good marks. On the other hand, I have a problem with questioning people even if they have much higher power levels than me. Sometimes I can become a bit intimidated and they take advantage of me. Other times I'll shoot my mouth off. If I disagree quite adamantly, I'll say so. I may be right, but it's the wrong way and the wrong time. I can be impulsive and do stupid things.

I like to know the reasons why. When material is presented or before a decision is made, I am constantly inquiring and trying to understand the reasons for a situation or process. Sometimes this makes people think I am argumentative. Other times they give me compliments on my enthusiasm. After I participated in a workshop that trained instructors to teach life saving techniques, the program designer approached me and told me I should be teaching the course. She had noticed that I talked my way through everything and explained why I was doing each step. She thought that would make me a really effective teacher. To me it was a necessary strategy. It's the only way I can learn and interpret the information. If you give me a sheet of paper full of information I can look at it, but if I don't go through the thought processes and reason why it's going on, I won't get it.

Sometimes I misunderstand people. I don't understand what they want. I can misinterpret questions on an exam or requests my mother makes. Some of these misunderstandings are easy to sort out, like making sure I have a written shopping list. Others are more complicated. I find I question myself. I feel unsure I am effectively communicating my ideas. I'm always wondering if my point is really getting across. It shakes my confidence. Some days I feel like I need to take an English course, or grab a dictionary to expand on what I'm thinking. I really admire people who can communicate their ideas well. Communication is fascinating to me.

By nature I am a terribly disorganized person, so I have become extremely organized because I realized that organization is the only way to get something out of mass confusion. I've learned to use structure. I get an outline, I get a process going and I'm set. The thing I get concerned about is the fact that it takes me a little bit of time to get that structure. Some of my friends can grasp the key ideas a little bit quicker. It takes me time to just understand the process, to read the question or the situation. I have to slow myself down so that I do understand. The specifics may take me longer, but I get the big picture. I may be slow at the front end, but when it comes to ideas I can blow most people off the map. I can just put the ideas flying down on paper. Then I'll just take a little bit of time to organize them and present them and hopefully we all reach the same endpoint together.

One of the major ways I cope with my learning disability is through athletics. I'm a rower. I do cross training with swimming, biking and running. Typically I would spend a minimum of three hours a day working out. My physical fitness allows me to cope with being hyper.

After a workout I can relax and get in about two or three hours of really good studying time. I've learned that physical activity and fun are directly related to me getting better marks. My stress gets released and it allows me to focus on the studying tasks at hand.

One of my heroes is Silken Laumann. She won a bronze medal at the 1992 Olympics for rowing. A few months before the competition, she was severely injured when the men's doubles boat from Germany crashed into her. She knew the odds of rowing in the Olympics were slim. She knew the odds of winning a medal were even smaller. No one except Silken knew her mental toughness or her determination. I see a parallel there with my own struggles. In my mind the key to my success in school and in life is a strong attitude, determination and a mind that can move around like a yo-yo.

Getting to University

One of my teachers in about grade seven noticed that there was something wrong. All through school, the teachers were always talking to my mother about my reading and writing. I have excellent mathematical skills. They just didn't match with the other things I was doing. Picture me as the kid who was always looking around and off in la-la land. We had a math teacher who played a game with us for drill. He would throw a basketball to the person who was supposed to answer the question. You were supposed to catch the ball, shout out the answer, and throw it back. I was the guy who was always getting beaned by the ball. I might have known the answer, but I sure couldn't play the game.

I was frustrated and my behaviour wasn't the best. I took my frustrations out at home. My family got frustrated. By the fall of grade ten, I was failing all five courses. One of my teachers gave me the benefit of the doubt and kept coming into class with different methods of dealing with the work. I managed to pull my marks up from 22 to 86 per cent in her class, but the rest of my life was pretty rough.

Basically, at that point in my life I was a frustrated, swearing person. I was failing. I was tripping over my own feet. I wasn't doing anything worthwhile and I just didn't feel right. I was seeing a psychologist for what might be termed weird behaviour. I was skipping classes at school and I had violent outbursts. I thought I knew everything and that no one understood. I was really frustrated with my parents for putting all this pressure on me. Pretty soon there was no one left. That's how I saw it.

Finally, I just lost it one night with my mom. I threw a chair at her, and wrecked half my room. I blew out of there and ran away to a neighbour's place down the street. I knew I had to leave home. I knew I had to slow down somehow and figure out what was going on. I had become violent with my mother. I thought, "This is pretty stupid! Something has got to change." That was a big turning point in my life. I started to understand that it was my problem.

I talked things over with my neighbour. She thought that there might be some medical problem. She knew that allergies affected the behaviour and emotions of some people. We went to the doctor and started to get things sorted out. It turned out that I did have allergies, particularly to codeine which I was taking. The doctor said, "Sure you may be frustrated, and have other problems, but there's an allergic reaction to a drug involved here. This is having a dramatic effect on your reaction to things." We figured that part out.

I met with my dad. We talked things over and then we went home to see my mother. My parents apologized for not knowing what was going on with me. They hadn't realized the nature of the attacks and the frustrations I was feeling. They saw that things were getting worse and worse, but they had been viewing things in the wrong way. They said they now understood what the psychologist and the doctor were talking about. They knew that we needed help and that we had to get to the bottom of all of this. They also said that I had to be responsible for myself. They sort of kicked me out into my own little world of being me. I agreed and I apologized. They forgave me and I came back home.

After that things started rolling in the right direction. My parents sent me to a children's centre for a psycho-educational assessment. It was there that I started to understand my disability problems and started to develop the skills to handle this stuff. My parents did too. I had to travel to the children's centre where they ran through a battery of tests with me for about three days. About a week after that, they called me in with my parents and explained what was going on. They offered some possible solutions. They explained to my parents what my behaviour would be in certain instances, and suggested ways my parents could deal with me to help relieve the stress when I was getting frustrated. They explained to me how to deal with certain actions and why I was acting in certain ways. They recommended remedial work and accommodations for school.

When I finally got all this testing done, it was paid for by my family. The school did not promote it. They recognized the problem, but they didn't actively get involved in having students diagnosed. For me, diagnosis was really important because it gave me a better understanding of my problems. Somebody else was actually confirming this. It was a relief to feel, "Maybe it's not just me!" Assessment identifies your weaknesses and it also points out things that you do better. I eventually just learned not to do the things that got me into trouble. Assessment was one of the most helpful things that happened to me.

After the assessment, I went to the special education class in my high school. They didn't call it that but I would. One of my eight courses was this special class. I was allowed to work on remedial reading, writing, artistic expression, and group discussion. Sometimes I worked with an individual teacher. Other times I was with a group. Basically we worked on skills that were a problem. I was around other students who had problems. Some were similar to mine and some were different. We all sort of helped each other out and that was how we learned.

The other big help was the de-stressor room. It was the place where I would be sent to cool off if I acted up in class. I could also just get up and go to that room if I was having problems in classes interpreting something and I was feeling really frustrated. I wrote all my quizzes and exams there too. I really needed adjustments at that school, but it was not until I had the assessment and diagnosis that adjustments were made for me that worked.

One of my best friends, Tim, has a learning disability too. His parents were really an amazing help to me all through this time. His mom and dad met on the third rewrite of an exam in a teacher training program. They struggled the whole way through school. It went right over their heads. They were taught one way and then they had to try six or seven different ways of teaching themselves. They were accepted into teacher training on personal recommendations rather than their academic records and they turned out to be great teachers. Former students still visit them. Whenever I had a problem understanding something, I'd take it to Tim's dad. He'd say he didn't understand it either, but we'd sit with his wife and bounce ideas around. Then they'd say this might be a way to work it and off I'd go with my problem straightened out.

Tim's parents were really effective in communicating ideas. They were great teachers and that's what Tim has learned. He is out west right now. Even though he is smart and a great communicator, he didn't make it through the university system. He rather enjoyed the partying and the social aspect of things, but university wasn't for him.

I would describe him as a very intelligent person, but not with a book. He's got social skills and communication down pat. He's teaching skiing now. He is doing well and enjoying himself. His father has gone off into administration. I feel it's a loss for students because he was such a good teacher. You remember key teachers in your life who have done a lot for you.

For grades eleven, twelve and thirteen, I switched to a private school. The classes weren't so large. I got more of the individual attention and feedback that I needed. There was an openness in the teachers that just wasn't there in my other high school. The teachers at the private school weren't the highest paid people, but they were very dedicated to the teaching process and they had special training for their jobs. They came in early and they stayed late. They gave you special help after class.

One of the key teachers taught English and I did really well in that class. Her course was feminist based and she loved Margaret Atwood. I found the course really interesting, but it always offended a bunch of guys in the class. I didn't take offense. I just figured that was her viewpoint. In my essays I would point out what I could agree with and then make an argument against the things I didn't agree with. The guys thought she wouldn't accept anybody's point of view but her own, and they just tried to toe the line. I was the only one who would stand up and challenge her. When I did, she would discuss why she had come to these conclusions, or compare one author with another. She would lead you down the path of her reasons. I figured out in her class that oral discussion really helped me to clarify and present my ideas. That's when I started to realize that getting picked on in class was a big help to me.

At the end of the year she made a speech, announcing that I had got the highest mark in the class. People in my class were shocked. Some of them said, "John you can barely write, for God's sake! How can you be getting the best mark in English?" Yes, that was true but she helped me learn. As far as she was concerned, learning was the point of the class. I could hand in a paper and she would show me the mistakes in spelling and grammar. We'd discuss the different points of view. I'd take it away and work on it again. It was a constant learning process. She didn't just mark it and hand it off. There was a constant cycle of feedback. That was the best thing about her. It really worked for me.

Feedback was stressed in that school. There were constant reports between my parents, me and the school. Frequent progress meetings were held that included both me and my parents. At first, I couldn't see the point in all of these meetings. They seemed pretty mundane. After a while I understood what was going on. Your parents were paying your way through school, so they were entitled to find out what you were doing. Were you in class? Were you learning the work? They'd go through all that but they also talked about what they were going to be teaching you and how they were going to teach it to you. They made suggestions about how parents could help at home and vice versa. We were all working together. It wasn't just me. It was sort of a three way street instead of a one way street. My marks went from the fifties to the eighties. Plus I enjoyed being at school with other people with learning problems. It was neat to be around the same sort of people who were having the same sort of general problems and had different ways of dealing with things.

At the beginning of school everybody is learning to cope with their learning style. Kids with ADD can do this too. This would be a great time to start. If you get students thinking they are special or out of the ordinary, it's not going to help anything. They may even think that they can use their special status to their advantage. I've seen kids use ADD as an excuse for everything, instead of just seeing that they have a different task or a hurdle to jump before they can do better.

After going through all of that, I feel that I am much more mature than most people of my age. I realize that if I'm not, I'm going to get right out of control. It wasn't always like that. Maturity of the individual is a key factor. I can see now that when you're younger, ADD interferes with the teaching environment. There are times when you've got to get the students with ADD out of the classroom and you've got to give them a way out that's not going to get them into trouble. I don't believe you should separate and isolate individuals with learning disabilities, or just send them through. The changes they made at high school gave me a way out and helped me learn to cope. You've got to allow students like me into the system. They have to learn to cope.

Next Stop University!
In the heat of the moment, I sometimes wanted to give up on marks and formal education no matter what school I was in. But I never really thought of dropping out. My parents have pretty high expectations for me and getting formal education was always part of that. My mother always made it clear that they would support me in getting an education. She also made it clear that they would not support me if I

just sat around the house. That was pressure I guess, but it also kept me motivated. My dad's philosophy is that if you see something that you'd like to be doing, try it. You can always try something else later, but don't miss the opportunity to learn about things you've never seen or tried before.

I want to do well for myself and to follow in the family tradition. My grandfather was a stockbroker who lost his job in the Depression. He owned a bakery after that to support his family and wound up doing very well. My father qualified as a carpenter and then went on to become an actuary. He too has done really well for his family. That's the way I would like my future to be.

I never questioned the idea of coming to university and staying there. It was just a question of which university to go to and how to learn as much as I could. With my learning disability, I knew that there was going to be a problem at university because of the time frames for exams, the increased level of difficulty and the pace of the work. I knew that I was going to have to come out with it and get some help, or I was going to flunk out. It was crucial that I found the place to study that would give me the best chance of succeeding.

In the spring of my final year in high school, my father and I toured all the schools that had accepted me. That way I could make a more informed decision about where to go. I got some first-hand ideas about what to expect and the chance to make some contacts for the fall. On one campus, I saw the high school liaison person who had made a presentation at my school. He saw me across the football field and welcomed me by name. I thought, "This school would be all right. It's a personal place." I figured if one of the recruiting officers who sees a couple of thousand kids can remember my name, then I'm sure the professors will know me, and understand my habits and my learning processes. There's a good chance that they will work with me and adapt. We can find a happy medium here. It turned out that my intuition was right. I made a good choice.

There were lots of challenges at university, but I just tried to learn from them and push the negatives aside. Some of this stuff you just have to ignore. If you dwell on the barriers and your miscalculations, you make them worse. I found that if I was worried about something and focused on it, the whole problem just increased tenfold. It would make everything bad and that was no solution.

My three best moments at university were getting in, graduating and going three for three at a rowing regatta. In all of these things, I had worked hard all season and then one day it all came together. The worst moment at university was in second year when I ran into a professor who was a complete roadblock. He bought my story about my learning disability and listened to my reasons for accommodation. Then he turned around and turned his back on me. He was the stereotype of the student's worst nightmare.

I thought the professor had agreed to let me write in a private setting with extra time. When I walked in to do the exam, he had decided that my concerns were irrelevant and I would have to write with everyone else. I had not planned for this or thought about how I would handle these conditions. When I'm not prepared and organized, my thoughts just won't come out even when I know the material. I couldn't walk away because I needed the course to get into my business program. I didn't know what else to do, so I sat there and tried to work on the exam. At the end of the allotted time, he took my paper away even though I hadn't finished, and told me I must be stupid not to be able to finish the test. He pointed out that there was another person in the class with a disability worse than mine, but she had finished in plenty of time.

This was really devastating. It was the big build-up period for the third year of the business program. This incident made me feel like I didn't have what it took to be at university. "I'm stupid. I must be, if I can't keep up with everyone else." What was really frustrating was that I had picked this professor especially for my learning style. I needed someone who would put notes on the board, explain things well, provide extra handouts and allow me to tape the classes. This professor was very good at all of that. He did a lot of questions on the board and he was very organized. In many ways he was an excellent instructor. The roadblock was his view of exam accommodations.

I was so frustrated that I came into the Counselling Centre in tears. I calmed down and went back to him later to discuss the issue. He would not do anything about that first exam. My mark was in the 60s. He thought I shouldn't be complaining, even if I felt it didn't reflect what I knew. He sent me away to try again on the next exam.

After intervention from the Counselling Centre, the professor agreed to let me write in private, with a few minutes of extra time. In the end, we had one misunderstanding after another. He was riled. I was riled. I was putting up a stink. Even with exam accommodation, my marks were going steadily down. I was helping other people in the class with the tough problems, but I could not do well on the exams. My classmates couldn't believe the marks I was getting since I was tutoring some of them. Math had always been a strength for me. The final grade was a composite of the four term exams. For two of those exams I had not received accommodation.

Fortunately, the contested course was a half-course that finished at Christmas. I was at home with my parents when I got my final mark. On the aggregate I fell three marks short of a passing grade. I had gone home in a really frustrated state of mind but after I got my marks, I was flipping mad. I talked with my parents and they were behind me. I also got some support from an alumnus living nearby, who had donated quite a bit of money to the school. I talked to my best friend's father who was a lawyer. He explained to me that there could be a lawsuit launched over this issue because it was discrimination. He was willing to provide his services for free if I wanted to proceed with a lawsuit. He felt he would enjoy making this kind of point to the education system. But what really did it was my dad saying, "We'll put the people behind you if need be. You have the backing to do whatever you want." All I really needed to know was that I had the support to pursue my point as far as I needed to.

I have always been taught to stand up and fight for myself. If you don't, you're done. I felt it would have been completely unfair for me to have to redo that course. It would also mean falling behind in my program requirements. I launched a formal appeal over the lack of accommodation and requested that my grade be changed to a pass. The whole appeal process was not an easy one, but it was better than not doing anything.

I came back after Christmas and spoke to my counsellor. We discussed the options and talked about formal and informal ways of working this out. She helped me understand the steps in the appeal process and helped me put together my case. I did formal and informal lobbying. I had always worked out every morning at the gym at the same time as the president of the university. I let him know how things were going. I took one little piece out of the system at a time. I wrote up my appeal letter and sent it in. I got letters of support and made sure they had all the necessary documentation.

The review process started a lot quicker than I expected. The professors on the appeal committee interviewed me separately. I felt they were really concerned and willing to listen to my side. Once that happened, I didn't see how I would fail. I didn't think that those people could honestly deny me a pass. They could see what I had done before and the accommodations I had used. I had worked hard and knew the material. Since I felt there were people on my side, I was able to just let it go and get on with the rest of the term.

One of the professors on the appeal committee was my instructor for a second term half course that year. He was great. He has a hearing disability himself. He caught on to the adjustments I needed right away. He said, "If you want to try my class to experiment, go right ahead." I wrote some tests in the classroom. I had extra time in a private setting for some. We tried different things. I understood his lectures. He made up special sheets for all of us to review. He was very flexible and interested in different ways of approaching problems. He seemed to enjoy looking at the different way I approached problems. He wasn't perfect and he didn't try to pretend that he was. When he made mistakes on the board, he was cool about it. We'd all laugh and start again. It got to the point where I could do the same work as everybody else and I wound up with an 80 in that course.

The irony is that the professor who didn't want to accommodate me had a disability too. He felt very strongly that disability shouldn't be used as an excuse. I agreed with him. It concerns me that some people could use their disability and the power it gives them to take advantage of the system, so I was never satisfied until I had put all the effort into a course that I could. But not giving students a chance to show that they know the material is a different issue. My learning disability may be a reason I don't understand something, but it's not an excuse. It just makes learning a different task, a hurdle to do better. My learning disability is something I have. I was born with it. You can't dwell on it, but it does come in handy to be able to explain to the professor the way that you think, and that there are certain situations where you can't understand or do the questions required. That is not using your disability as an excuse.

Throughout this appeal process, there was a lot of frustration. I tried to make things in my life more positive. De-stressing was really important. I wasn't going to give up! I would go out with my friends and do little things that made me feel good. I kept up my physical activities. I found the people around me who were supportive and talked to them. There were the counselling services at the school, close friends, my family and other professors who knew that I was a good student. I found out what I was worth from all of that. Going out with my friends and doing physical activities allowed me to go back, recoup, hit the books and try again.

In the end the departmental appeal committee acted quickly and granted me a passing grade. Was it worthwhile? It was tough. I'd say it took an average amount of energy to understand and explain the different issues involved. The actual writing of the appeal, the organizing and presenting of it, took a lot of time. Because this involved the professor's reputation I wanted to be really careful. This could have serious consequences for him. I didn't feel that he should be kicked out of school for this. In fact I felt he was an excellent teacher. It wasn't his teaching that was a problem. It was his refusal to accommodate me. I thought that was the key issue to focus on. Bringing the key issues out was difficult, but I had lots of help in the end. Appealing was easier than just sitting there and saying, "I've got an extra course to do this term. Great! How am I going to pull this off?"

Now when I look back, I think of that appeal as a critical point. It had a huge influence on me. Coming to university, I didn't feel that I had much power or control over things. I was just some student. This incident taught me about power. I discovered I had resources and I discovered how to use them. I learned about how careful you have to be in using power. You don't want somebody having power without understanding the influences and repercussions of misusing it.

The whole thing taught me to trust myself and my instincts. I didn't get this far without a reason. I learned how to present my case. I had enough support and trust in people to do it. It gave me confidence in myself and it gave me confidence in the system. These professors made a fair and honest decision in favour of a student. Thankfully, I never had to go the appeal route again but I knew that if I had to, I could.

Learning at University

I have to try to adapt my learning style to the demands of each situation. At university, lectures are a really useful part of my learning time. I process vocal and visual information much more quickly than I do from simply reading and writing something. I take notes quite poorly. In lectures I have to concentrate more on what the professor is saying than taking notes. I do have my own style of taking notes using colour coding, but when professors use overheads I try to pick up copies of them. I make sure I pick up copies of questions that are assigned and any answer sheets or outlines that are available. I like to have this written material for reference to make sure I have understood and have all the details.

Because of the way I process vocal information, I can record a professor's lecture in my head. When my friends come to me after a class and ask me what the professor said here or there, I can recite it back to them. I find this ability especially useful and it is a kind of bargaining tool in getting me proper notes. I tell them what was said in class and they lend me notes. We switch back and forth like that.

I find that I have peak learning times. Six o'clock in the morning to five o'clock at night is good. The first hour or two after I exercise is best. Anytime, after five o'clock my brain shuts off. I don't know what it is. This makes evening classes or project meetings a real challenge. I schedule to avoid them if I can.

For exams, I need accommodation. I find that I have to sit down in a quiet, private space and read the exam out loud to myself. If I just read the exam silently, I have absolutely no understanding of the question. By reading aloud, it slows me down and I can draw out the points of the question. Sometimes I hand my answers in to the proctor one question at a time so that I don't get my rough notes mixed up and lose track of my organized ideas. Depending on the type of question I may use flipchart paper and coloured markers to help me get my ideas out and organized. Then I read my answers into a dictaphone. This seems to slow my thoughts down and I get my answers transcribed from the tape for the professor to mark. Other times I use a computer, which is faster and clearer than writing.

One of the problems I find with a subject like accounting is that the questions become very broad as you progress. They take in a whole bunch of different concepts. With a broad question I can't always orient myself to decide which six points I am supposed to respond to. If I am writing in a private setting, I can't just raise my hand and ask if the professor would clarify the question a bit, or confirm that I have understood and am on the right track. That is the trade-off in writing away from the class. I have found that some of my professors have been very good about checking in with me, wherever I am writing, to give me a chance to clarify any of the questions that are puzzling to me.

For classes, I find the professor's presentation skills and approach extremely important. I find it very helpful if the professor gives me some visual information: overheads, writing on the board, lecture notes. The best style for me is a professor who repeats the ideas. Someone who says this is the job we are going to do today, talks about it and then summarizes. In that way I get the information three times and I get the general drift of the lecture. The input may be a little bit disorganized, but there is time to work on that after class.

After the first couple of classroom sessions, I discuss with professors my willingness to answer questions in class. This puts the onus on me to be prepared, to focus and to understand the material. My major motivation for doing this is that I feel really stupid if a professor asks me a question and I don't know the answer. I will work very hard not to be embarrassed in front of my peers. I find this way I can use my relationship with my peers as a motivator.

Discussion in class really helps me a lot. I enjoy the dialogue and I can demonstrate to the professor that I understand the material. I am often more successful at doing this in a vocal way than I am when I am writing on paper. This makes me feel more secure at exam times. If I make a mistake or really get off track in the exam, the professor realizes that I actually know the material and we can sort something out.

A detailed outline of the structure of the course is critical for me. This is usually pretty standard practice. I find it gives me a timeline to follow. I need a plan and an overview. I can budget for my busy times and I can figure out a logistic scheme to cope with the load. I can build in breaks to keep me going. I may need support from other people to stay organized, or to reorganize my plan when something has gone wrong, but I have to have a structure to start with. Along with the structure, it is really important to have someone you can rely on to talk to when things go wrong.

At university I've never worried about getting high marks. You have to maintain a certain standard in order to stay on and graduate, so I wanted marks enough to pass, but I've had to find other ways of motivating myself. I use marks as a signal to judge if I understand the course. They are another way of getting feedback. A seventy-five can be cause for a good night out. An eighty-five can be cause for a great weekend. A fifty tells you to slow down and look again.

Marks can be a good management tool. They can drive you forward, but they can also be a big source of frustration if you are learning disabled. What's more important to me is to ask, "What did I personally get out of the course? What did I learn?" Some of the best classes I've had, in terms of enjoyment and the learning aspect, haven't been my best classes in terms of marks. Some marks are a real source of satisfaction. The best marks are the ones you feel you've really earned with a combination of good effort and good learning.

I had to learn pretty early on to make the distinction between the mark you get and what you know. When I was in grade eight, my marks weren't all that great and they told me I was writing at the grade four level. I thought, "Well, I've got this far. I must be doing something else right that teachers are interested in because they keep passing me.

I guess marks aren't all that important." So I just carried on learning for myself.

My mother would nag me about marks. She was constantly telling me that I needed good marks to get to university, or to do anything. To her, they were an essential aspect of my education and proof that I understood my work. My father was more low key about marks. He supported my mother, but he had a different attitude to learning. He told me "I don't care what marks you get. It's what you learn that counts. It's the process of learning that is important. Go to university. Do all of your class work, but most importantly find out what you have missed. Do that all the time. Those are the qualities you need for the real world. You want the real world skills, not just book smarts. Sometimes it may feel like you have to tie both your feet together and try walking, but you can still get to where you want to go. If the only way you learn is to trip, that's okay as long as you learn from your mistakes. It's just a little bit different. There are enough people in the world with book smarts and we've got the computer now for all of those facts and details."

For my children, I want them to know that marks are important. I want them to do well in school, but the most important thing is the process of learning. I want them to be actively involved and able to use what they have learned. I would always ask them if they had put in a good effort. If they said they had, I wouldn't worry about the mark. Sure, good marks make a person happy, but I want my children to be happy because they've done the work and they are well prepared.

You Remember the Teachers

Most professors I've had at university didn't have a problem with my learning style. Some of them have been very encouraging in their own ways. I found that professors have different styles, not only in the way they present material, but also in the way they deal with me. I didn't always need to have the same style of professor. I've learned how to respect the professors for their strengths and weaknesses and how to figure out what they had to teach me.

Even though I prefer teachers who are informal, all I need is a professor who is willing to establish a dialogue with me about the course. We can negotiate from there. Feedback is how I learn and professors are an invaluable source of feedback. I need lots of feedback, the more direct the better. I don't care if my argument gets ripped to shreds. I need to know what I'm missing. Most of my professors were really willing to help me once they understood that I wasn't challenging them, criticizing their teaching, or trying to get out of work.

A student's approach to starting this dialogue is really important. I learned through trial and error how to have a discussion about the material without appearing to question the professor's judgment or to be scraping for more marks. I think the secret was focusing on the learning process and establishing that I was willing to do the work to fill in the gaps in my knowledge. I used questions like: What did I miss? What are the key issues? How could I do better? Sometimes it can seem almost impossible to find out how you can do well in the course, but if you've established a dialogue with the professor and a feeling of mutual respect at least you can keep trying.

One of my professors was always encouraging me to battle it out with him. I'd get really frustrated with him when he wouldn't allow me all of the accommodations that I was requesting. Then I realized that this was his challenge to me. He wanted me to do well. He was always pushing me to get into the mainstream. I enjoyed his classes. He was humorous and a good communicator. I felt I learned a lot, even if I wasn't getting the best marks, so I kept on trying. Then when I had finally shown him what I could do, he said, "Okay, you've convinced me. I understand now." He readjusted the weighting of the course evaluations, and allowed me credit for class participation and individual tutorial work with him. Personal dialogue and negotiations with a professor who is very traditional and oriented to the mainstream, but wants to help you, can be very rewarding. It can also be very difficult and emotionally challenging. If it works out well, you can wind up with a real sense of accomplishment.

Another one of my professors took much more of a supportive, counselling role. A family experience with learning disabilities had made him familiar with the situation. I could talk easily to him and he always made me feel that I could do well in his course. He said I could try different things and make a challenge out of his course. The first term was a half course. I got through okay, but he suggested that I shouldn't take the second term of advanced work. Given the nature of the course, he didn't think I would do well. I said, "I don't care what you think. I love this course. I want to take the second half. I don't care if I fail. The marks aren't what I'm here for. I want to learn the process and understand what goes on."

The professor saw my point and got behind me. He gave me extra help. He'd talk to me after class and give me an hour or so every week of his own time to discuss the material. He would make sure I understood what was going on. He found people in the class for me to talk to about the problems. He gave me practice problems with model answers plus a checklist of topics. After all the exams, I would go over and discuss what I had done and explain how I reasoned through the problems. It got to the point that I could do the same work as everyone else even though I might do it differently. In the end, I got the credit.

I found that course very difficult. I worried about it the whole time. I knew I wasn't able to keep pace in understanding the material. I've had that happen before. If you think of the course as a river, I've got a dam system in place, backing things up. The river won't flow and neither will my answers. I got 44 in the mid-term, but then things started flowing and I wound up with a 60. I felt like I had walked through fire.

Another professor I admired adopted a friend and mentor role with me. I really enjoyed working with him. I felt there was mutual understanding and respect. I met him when he was proctoring my exam for another professor. He gave me the wrong exam. It was one he had for his own class. I looked at the questions and they were things I had never seen before. I thought, "Oh, boy! What have I done this time?" I couldn't see anything I'd studied for, but I thought I must have messed up on my studying and missed the stuff the professor decided to put on the exam. I gave it my best shot anyway. I sat there for about four hours puzzling my way through the questions. Luckily, I had extra time.

Once I got out of the exam and started talking to other students from my class, I realized what had happened. I had been given the wrong exam. I went back to the professor who had proctored the exam and he offered to let me write the test with him in his office while he marked his exams. I liked the idea of getting it over with while my studying was still recent, but I was too frustrated to do it. I took the exam, but I didn't know what the hell I was doing and I let it show. When I hadn't settled down after a few minutes, he sent me out to run around the track and have some lunch. Then we started over. He marked the paper I had written for his exam and on that one I got the second highest mark in the class. I had done really well on the problems. The only thing I hadn't aced was the technical definitions. We became great friends after that.

Later on I took one of his courses. He was very encouraging. He thought a person didn't have to follow just one orthodox method to learn. He said he had been self-taught and he showed me how I could learn to teach myself. He taught me how to approach a problem from different angles. He gave me backup strategies to use to interpret the problems. He didn't focus on micro-solutions and let me suit my learning style. I always seemed to find it easier to go backwards from the answer into the problem, so he would put the answer at the bottom of the page and work backwards with me. I was able to focus on the key issues when I started at the end of the sequence. That way I wouldn't get lost in the details of the problem and I could do the hardest part of the problem, the reasoning. Once I got the method down, I could start from either end.

Teamwork and Friends

I like working as part of a team. I like the contact and the feedback. You talk things out and share ideas. You can balance the work off and cover for one another. There are some things I just can't do. Some people may see that as freeloading at first. Usually, after I explain and they see me contributing my share, it's not a problem. I always start off getting people to talk about their learning strengths and joking around about what you do well and what you don't. It's a good networking skill. It helps the group get to know one another. Often I wind up being the group leader because I'm good at analyzing the tasks, organizing the process and delegating. The business program often uses team projects and I've really enjoyed them. I wish we'd had more of them. I love trying to apply the things we've been studying and putting together a project. It gives me a real sense of accomplishment. The presentations are scary, but it's great when people come up to you afterwards and say, "Hey, you really convinced us." I usually get compliments like that and good marks on my presentations.

When the team works it's great, but the down side of being different is that you always have a different point of view. Sure it can make you a really valuable part of the team, but it can sometimes get annoying. I might start questioning myself when there are a bunch of ideas floating around, "Why didn't I think of that? I shouldn't be here!" Sometimes people don't take your answers seriously and give them much credit. They just walk over them. On one or two occasions I've had the whole group against me. I've explained and explained my point, but I couldn't convince them. I remember this, because in the class the professor agreed with my point of view. I tried with the group, but there's not always much you can do.

I have found it really useful to develop study teams. It gave me a great opportunity to make some really good friends at the same time as I was getting my work done. Sometimes I teamed up with someone from my class. Other times it was someone who just loved to discuss things, or whose interests and skills complemented mine.

One of my buddies was another student with a learning disability who was a couple of years ahead of me. He was someone I could look up to and learn from, but he was also someone like me and someone I could help out. He was hopeless at reading and writing things down, but he was the best person with a dictaphone. Things just needed to be oral for him. If you read him what you had written for your paper, he could critique it and discuss the argument with you. We'd have this exchange and I'd find better ways of developing and backing up my argument. I would do the same for him.

One time in residence, this same friend and I were ordering pizza with some of the guys. They gave him a written list of what they wanted. I went to the phone with him and heard what he ordered. When the food arrived, it was nowhere near what anybody had ordered. They kept going through the food saying, "Who ordered this?" and no one would claim the stuff. So my friend says, "Hey, why are we surprised? We're learning disabled. I can't read and he can't listen. Next time either yell out the order to me, or write it down for him." Everybody laughed and started eating. It would have been very different for me if I'd been in that situation alone.

This year, my friend is working at the university as a resource educator in the program for students with disabilities. As part of his job he would be available to work with me on my projects. The funny thing is it doesn't work the same way for me now. He's still a great guy, but it's just not the same as working along with someone like you. I used to see him almost every day. Now that he's not a student, he's around at different times. Mainly, what I think I missed was the encouragement his attitude as a student gave me. I'd look at him trying to write a paper and I'd think, "It's never going to happen. He'd be as likely to build a rocket launcher." But he always got it done. It gave me the sense of working together with somebody in the same boat. He was a mentor and a friend. He'd make fun of my learning disability and I'd make fun of his. It made things better.

This past year, I've tried to do things more on my own. My courses have been more formal. My classmates are all busy competing for jobs. I feel like we are all competing, even in class. Some of my mentors have moved on. I have really missed that sense of working together. It makes school a lot harder for me. Working partners are both a resource and a motivator for me.

Managing my Energy

So I have ADD! The world is moving to a multi-task state. What do I do best? High energy, multiple tasks, multiple ideas. I am a person born at the right time. I can get people going with my energy when they are dead tired. I can keep a rowing crew going when they think there's nothing left. I can use my energy to pull people along and inspire them. I don't look at my learning disability as being a problem anymore.

What I have to watch out for, is that I will burn out. When I do crash, get out of my way! There is that side of me and I have to be careful. Once I learned about my disability, I started to learn how to manage my energy. One of the worst things that ever happened in my life was that period of violent outbursts. I promised myself I would never be violent again.

I've spent a lot of time thinking about the skills I need to manage my energy. I know I can use physical exercise to keep myself under control. Eating properly helps. I have to watch my stress level. I feel high as a kite after a workout, but I am also at my most relaxed. I feel clear-headed and I can get all kinds of things done. I like to be busy. I like to be doing something or I'm bored out of my tree. Ever since I was a kid, I was always doing things around the house. I loved doing painting, repairs, lawn-care and whatever my dad could come up with. I enjoyed building things and doing models too. I liked being able to see the results of my work and I liked the sense of accomplishment it gave me. I felt useful because I had done something.

When I came to university and was trying to figure out how to handle my time without getting totally stressed out, one of my buddies suggested that I should work as hard as I could for six days and then take a day off. I tried that system, but I couldn't stand it. That day off was the most frustrating day of my week. I found out that I had to be doing some school work every day, or I was really uncomfortable. The routine keeps me going. I decided I just had to pace myself. I would work every day and then, once a month have a big get-away break. I'd set my goals first, then when I had accomplished them, I was off for a big treat. I think I inherited that kind of work style from my dad. He always likes to be busy and keep on top of things. Every once in a while, he finds a relaxing activity and takes a break. That seems to work for me too.

Sometimes my energy can get in the way in my relationships. I can generate excitement and enthusiasm, but I also need to cool down. I had one impulsive relationship with a girlfriend, idiot that I am. Now I know what the pitfalls are. I've met someone new and I know how to stay the course. We talk about what's going on. I know what to do and she does too. I tell her what cools me out. If we get into an argument, I just pick her up, throw her over my shoulder and run up and down the stairs. She just stays there and laughs at me the whole time. By the time I'm done, I've calmed down and burned up a lot of energy. She's had a good laugh and says, "All right, let's start arguing again." By that time, I've probably forgotten about the argument, or at least it doesn't seem the same and we deal with it. We both have developed skills to handle the situations that cause problems.

It's not just my energy that interferes. The way my memory works is a big issue too. I can forget what someone said to me ten seconds ago, but I will remember it the next day. I've got this twelve-hour delay in my head while I process what went on. I can comprehend things a little bit later on, but I have to take a little bit of time to think things out. Remembering specific details of lists or directions is just not going to happen. If I jot things down I can organize myself, but I have to do it right away because small details go right over my head. Sometimes it's because I am focusing on something else at the time, though it's not always obvious that I'm not getting what's going on. Going for groceries or running an errand without written instructions is a recipe for frustration for both me and the person I'm supposed to be helping out. If my girlfriend wants me to do an errand, she knows there are two steps. She has to put it down on paper and then tell me what she wants.

For work at my summer job in a greenhouse, my girlfriend gave me a little notepad to stick in my back pocket. I needed to have a quick reference to keep track of my duties for the day and some points on gardening at my fingertips. I can't call them up from memory on the spot. When someone mentioned something for me to do, I'd jot it down. If someone was knowledgeable about a certain topic in gardening, I'd write down that information. Later when someone asked me a question I could say, "I know that. It's right here in my book." It was great! The stress disappeared. I always had the security of knowing everything was in my book.

In my last year at university I wasn't really stressed out. I worried about the usual things, exams and graduating, but basically I was okay. The thing is, my mind can play tricks on me. Sometimes I crash and feel hopeless, or sometimes I can set my mind to something and get it done no matter what. I get bursts of energy and I go through cycles.

It's a question of recognizing what point I'm at in the cycle and working with it.

The problem with me is that life is either great or rock bottom. I usually hit rock bottom about twice a year. That's when I just have to get away from it all and take a break. I'm usually pretty good at finding the support I need once I crash. Last time this happened, I found it really helpful just to talk it through with someone. After I did that, I started to see that I've worked hard and it will count. I've paid my dues, done my work and that will influence things falling my way. I don't have to hang onto the past, or worry about the future. I was able to settle down and get on with things. That's what I have to do.

The Long View, with Short Term Goals

Keeping perspective and setting goals is really important for me. I've developed what I call a long view of the world with a short-term perspective. That's how I operate. I set long range goals, middle range goals and short-term goals. A short-term goal might be, "How can I plan my day today?" I've got to set goals and set my mind to have things happen. I'm lost without that structure. Some of this I learned from the management tools in my business program, but I'd say rowing really brought home to me the strength of that approach. When you work on rowing with a coach, you work from a planned work out. You can see right from the start how things will go week by week. You focus on a few things at a time and you test it. You use the feedback you get to keep building toward the planned goal. You can always see where you are and where you are going.

This past summer I decided I was going to get to the big national rowing regatta. The whole situation was ideal for me. My day job was working at the greenhouse where I was both active and relaxed. For training, I was part of a crew with a good coach and the commitment to get there. We'd race on Saturday and get together in the evening to relax. Then on Sunday, we'd get up to go for a long row and experiment. We'd try out different things to see if we couldn't get better. After that workout we'd be pretty tired, but instead of going away to recuperate, we'd all sit around together having breakfast and discussing what we did and what to try next. We'd have Monday off and then start the cycle again.

That's what I like about rowing. You are essentially doing the same thing over and over again, but there are 367 things that can go wrong with a stroke. There's constantly something to work on. There are all these different champions with their theories. They tell you how they think, how they motivate themselves and what you look like to them. Nothing's ever perfect. There's constant feedback. "I think you're doing that wrong. Try this!" It's a constant learning process. I feel great after a really long workout on the water and I love just sitting around yapping about the whole process.

We did get to the regatta and that was our goal. We knew we weren't likely to win anything, but getting there was our aim and we did it. All kinds of things happen at a big regatta. That year a team of professional football players decided to compete. They had never rowed before, but they decided to put a boat in the water to see what they could do. They made a decent showing and got a round of applause from all of the other competitors. The Canadian team lost to the Americans by a bow length. Given their best recorded times to that point, the Canadians should have been blown away. They should have lost by about seven boat lengths. The American team was so impressed that they stood up at the end of the race and gave the Canadians an ovation. I love stories like that, where the mind conquers the body. It proves to me that by following your goals and your vision, your mind can take you where you want to go, even if it is against the odds. I think that's what I've done at university.

Future Plans

I've always had an itch to teach things. My two major jobs, at the pool and at the greenhouse, have involved teaching. At the greenhouse, I enjoyed helping the customers and sharing with them what I'd learned about gardening. I was constantly on the move, which was good for me, but the contact was pretty limited. Teaching swimming was much more rewarding. It's really satisfying to teach kids something they didn't know before. You are left to teach on your own. You use all the creative ideas you have. If that still doesn't work you can tap your buddies on the shoulder and see what they are doing with their groups. You watch out for each other. You have to be aware of everything going on around. You've got to be able to calmly communicate alarms and react quickly to do your part if there's an emergency. Sometimes the parents might flip out about something, but other times when the kids have done really well the parents might take the whole staff out to dinner. I realize I can't teach swimming forever, but I really enjoy that job.

Ideally, I'd like to be self-employed. I'd like to do something in the rowing industry. I've got a lot of creative ideas and designs and I've got the motivation to put it through. I've been told this by my crews and people at the rowing club. They have been really encouraging, but I don't have access to capital. I don't have financial stability just yet. I'm holding these ideas in reserve for the time when I have the basics, like a roof over my head and food on the table. Then I can make a gentleman's bet, as they say, and try some of these things. I might do stupid, crazy things, but I've got this really conservative background that is a stabilizing force for me. At first my parents had to provide a strong, strict outline, otherwise I'd be off. That was part of their role, but I think I'm at the point now where they've done all the grounding they can. Now I've got to get out and do it myself.

In planning for the future, I think part of what I have to do is to ignore some of the frustration that my mom and dad have had. I'm dealing with different things. You can't basically give your parents the bird and walk away. They're putting the roof over your head. They're paying for your education. They are being extremely good to you. They really want me to have a professional degree and some financial stability so that I can choose from among some better options. I like that idea too, but I want to find out what job is really right for me first. I don't want to walk straight into another training program to get a professional designation.

When I came back to school for my final year, I was all set and hyper to get a chartered accountant job. I was signing up for all of the interviews. Then I realized after going through a couple of them, this is just an aristocratic process. Both the interviews and the jobs seemed like that. I saw big bureaucracy. I would be assigned a specialized skill and learn a specialized formula. I wouldn't have the big picture of how things operate. I wouldn't be able to work out with the clients how to match the math and accounting tools that I've gained with the skills they need. The whole philosophy and competitiveness was putting me right off. It wasn't for me. So I said, "Enough of that! I'm not worrying about jobs until I graduate. I'm not worrying about anything else until I get through. I have to set my priorities."

I do things differently. I have to do things differently. This past year I tried to write one or two exams under the same conditions as everyone else with a few others in the professor's office. I was trying to prove to myself that I could get more main stream, but I realize now that I don't stand a chance. I've got to do things in my own way, the way that least frustrates me. It's the only way that works for me. I have to really work to convince my parents on this one.

I would be happier following my instincts, and doing volunteer work to get a better idea of the people and processes involved in business jobs. I've noticed at school that I don't do well in the first set of exams at mid-term. It's not that I haven't studied. It's just that I don't have an understanding of the people and the process of the course. I need more information. If I'm volunteering, I'm getting experience and learning how to read people and situations. People are going to be much more willing to answer my questions and help me out if it's a volunteer experience. I'm not getting paid. I'm giving them a service, so I'm paying for the feedback. Then I can apply what I've learned in other situations and have a better idea what job's best for me. I think I understand my learning disability about 80 per cent now. The rest I'm going to have to sort out by working.

Right now I want to earn some money and put a roof over my head. I can always teach swimming. I can go back to the greenhouse business for the summer. They are willing to let me help out with the accounting and learn the system this year. I really enjoyed some of the sociology, philosophy, and political science courses I took as options. They were a change from business, but I also liked the aspect of looking more into society and human nature. They gave you more of an understanding of yourself and I found that useful. I was thinking I might take some more courses for interest. I could see if my mother could set me up with some volunteer work in some of the shelters and groups she's involved with. And then there's rowing! I've got some definite goals for rowing and a coach that can take me there. Basically, I'd like to go it on my own and see what happens.

Success

I feel like I've been successful. I'm happy with what I've done here and I think that's all that really matters. I think this school and this community did wonders for me. It taught me a lot about myself. I found I didn't have to be all school, business and marks. I am more people-oriented anyway. I found much more happiness in working with my friends discussing school, rather than just sitting down behind a desk pounding away at numbers and theories and all of that. This was a big change for me. At home I always moved around in schools, so I've only had a few close friends. I never felt part of a community with a wide variety of friends and a party network. Here at university I stayed with my old style and developed a few close friends, but I also knew a whole bunch of people that I could count on. That was different and that's what I liked. My friends were as close as the ones that I had at home, but I had fifteen or twenty people that I knew through classes that were much closer than my classmates back home. I found them more supportive and I found counting on people a little bit easier. That's what I liked. Here I didn't just rely on someone else to solve my problems. I learned to stick up for myself and work together with others. What happened to me fits with the philosophy of the institution about social justice and community building.

Am I successful compared to everybody else? Sure, I'm graduating with everybody else. I'd say I'm about average in terms of marks, but as I've learned before, that doesn't really tell you anything. I think it's what you have learned about yourself and about the people around you that counts. That's what you're supposed to take away. In those terms I certainly feel that I've been a success.

THE VIEW FROM OUTSIDE

John is a very impressive young man. He is extremely bright and personable. He has success written all over him. What I didn't know at our first meeting was how hard won that success was, or the high price he would continue to pay to complete his university education. John introduced himself to me as a person with attention deficit disorder. He was the first student with that formal diagnosis that I had encountered at university. Both his intelligence and his energy were readily apparent, but his disability was not. John had a very winning manner. He was pleasantly business-like, with an eagerness and self-deprecating sense of humour that shone through. He could discuss his learning style and he had clear goals for his education and career. He already seemed to be an effective self-advocate.

John and his father had arranged a pre-admission scouting tour of eligible universities. They arrived at my door with documentation describing John's learning disability and a set of questions about our programs. Past experience had shown them that John had the potential to be either a 30 or an 80 per cent student, so he and his parents were doing everything possible to ensure that he found a university environment where he had a chance for success. They had travelled from an urban centre where they had used resources and support systems to good effect. Judging from John's conversation and his accomplishments, their plans and strategies had been working well. His graduating average from high school was 82 per cent and he had a lengthy list of school and community activities along with his academic achievements. For me, as a service provider, these two were a joy to meet. They were doing everything a good practitioner might recommend and they were making it look easy.

In fact, many school and life situations were not easy for John. His mind moves quickly and he often isn't able to keep track of essential details. The speed and scatter of his attention result in some chaotic daily living experiences. He doesn't always understand the changing social context of his environment. Sometimes his intentions and need for assistance have been mistakenly interpreted as aggressive or demanding. To a casual observer, he might appear to be a guy who was more interested in going to the gym and working out than studying, but these activities were an essential part of his study regime. Rather than use medication, John used exercise and time management to work with his attention deficit. He did not enjoy the side effects of taking medication, but he enjoyed all kinds of sports and excelled at swimming and rowing.

John carries an incredible energy field. When focused it is a thing of beauty, but I can tell you that the room where he wrote his exams looked shaken with the strain of containing him. He seemed to have a physical impact on the space. There were periods in most days when he could not function well. He was able to recognize those periods and had the discipline to work when it was possible. The strength and determination he exerted to control and focus his energy was remarkable. Excelling in some aspects of his life provided John with the strategies for handling his weaknesses and the confidence to do things differently. His self-awareness and resilience allowed him to balance the pain and frustration of his disability with humour, generosity of spirit and some very creative strategies.

John has a vision of his own success and his place as part of a family that has experienced difficulties and transformed them into opportunities. They all believe that a setback is not the end of the road, but a natural part of the process of living and learning. John is willing to work hard and fight for his success even when it is challenged by an uncooperative professor or the barriers presented by his own learning style. Under the stress of deadlines or conflict, he may still be thrown back emotionally to those early school failures where he felt stupid, hopeless and frustrated, but he now understands this in a different way. He sees this flood of negative feelings as a phase of his work cycle associated with fatigue and takes steps to get through it. At times like that, he knows he needs a friendly presence to help him refocus. Sometimes he came to the counselling center for "de-stressing," but we weren't always necessary.

What became evident to me over the time that I worked with him was his willingness to use the techniques and feedback that he gathers from a whole range of people. Teaching, intervention and support from parents, friends and professionals had made a big impact on his life. He was still applying the lessons he had learned from the teachers in his life who had made a difference to him. He applied the principles of the physical lessons he learned from rowing and swimming, where he excelled, to help him become a better student. Even those 'mundane' meetings that someone at his school must have insisted he attend as a teenager had helped him understand effective strategies. John is constantly learning, reframing and refocusing in order to carry on and succeed. He is able to profit from all kinds of situations, even those that might look like disaster to someone who was not determined to succeed. I have heard the Olympic athletes that John admires say that this is the true sign of a champion.

Throughout his life, John has been able to draw support and inspiration from people around him who recognize and value his will to learn and excel. I have seen him mentor younger students with learning disabilities, and speak to groups of teachers and parents to help them keep on trying. I know he wants to be like those people in his past who made a critical difference for him. At graduation, in his typical style, John had generated a wealth of good ideas about what could come next for him. Getting settled in a new environment and sorting out the details of daily living will be a big challenge, but whatever comes his way you know that John will be brave in trying.

7
JOHN CARPENTER
World of Work

I met with John at a quiet café among the towers of the financial district in London. He had just flown into the United Kingdom for a business meeting the next day. We took advantage of his evening off to put together some thoughts on his life since university. In the midst of a demanding schedule his manner still conveyed a warm, easy competence and an enthusiasm for the task of sharing his experiences. He clearly valued the opportunity to help other people with the challenges of a learning disability and balancing the demands of career and family. Here are his reflections.

What Stays with You

After forty years of living, lots of questions occur to me when I think about where I am now and how I got here. What are you constantly dealing with on a day-to-day basis? What gets worse? What gets better? What skills do you still bring across and use? How do you find and develop new ones? What are the secrets to it? What do you learn about yourself? Then, because I have a young family, what are some little tips and tricks that might be helpful for others dealing with family relationships?

I know my learning disability is still there but it doesn't impact me as much. I'm more in tune with myself so the way that I learn isn't as disabling. I catch on to what's happening to me and I recognize the signals in my life much more quickly as I have gotten older. I guess you could say my learning disability doesn't cause me to sway off course as much. I think I retrained my body and developed skills that I didn't quite realize that I had. These strategies are part of me and the way I operate now. The vast number, maybe ninety-five percent, of the coping skills I use today are the ones I learned when I was young. On the surface they may change as you adapt to new circumstances but basically, they are the same. I know that certain things challenge me. It's been a journey of trying to figure out: What do I have in my back pocket that I can use when I need to? What do I need to work on? Now I have a family and a career in business but I am still searching and always trying to make things better.

How I Got Here

Following university, I had a number of business-related jobs but nothing I really wanted to stay with. I also tried coaching rowing at a boys' school but that definitely wasn't for me. After about three years I decided it was time to change my situation. I have family ties in the United Kingdom so I applied to university there to study for a master's degree in business administration (MBA). I knew that I still had attention difficulties and learning issues but I was just three years out of university. I thought the skills I needed for studying were all still fresh in my mind. The first thing that hit me was that I was not learning as fast as I used to. I didn't pick up information like I did before. It seemed like I had lost the ability to memorize. I'm never much of a student of the book. I'm terrible at reading academic papers. I find them boring. I can't seem to understand the material. I usually just look at the abstract or the first part of a study and go from there. In the MBA program that wasn't enough.

I'm a student of life so I looked at some of my former exam papers to see what I had written. When I actually looked at the questions, my answers were very practical. I found out for myself that I pick up what I'm seeing. My learning style is to see pictures. I see words spoken with pictures to remember situations and information. I am reminded of that again now when I'm studying German. That awareness had kind of slipped away from me.

With my job selling insurance I had picked work that was all oral. I was always on the phone and it suited my strengths. It was an intuitive choice. I didn't realize the strategy I was constantly using. It had become automatic. Then I came back to university and back into a medium of books. Funny thing, I was back to square one. But I didn't stay there. I adjusted as best I could. I used my old strategies and a few new ones. Case studies and competitions were great for me. I was an award winner but I won't say it was easy convincing them to award me my degree.

I moved on to work with a multi-national firm in Switzerland. At first, I was pretty lost in my new environment but that's how I met my wife. She helped me find my way back to my new apartment. It's an interesting story. On my first week I was invited to a party by some people from the office. It was outside of the city. I went but I thought I should leave early to make sure I didn't miss the public transportation link. One of the other guests offered me a ride home with her friends so I could stay on and enjoy the evening. The funny thing was, after we all piled into the car and arrived in the city, all I could remember about where I lived was my address and a big distinctive sign on a store in my neighbourhood. I knew my stop on the public transport but that was it. None of this meant anything to them and I didn't have any sense of where I was in the city. We tried asking a bus driver and a few pedestrians that were out as late as we were but no one could help. Finally, my wife came up with the idea of calling a cab and giving them the address. It worked and the next day I called to invite her out for a coffee in appreciation. I was interesting enough for her to accept a date and eventually my proposal of marriage. I still work and live with my family in Switzerland. I've changed firms, roles and projects over the years but my career has gone pretty well.

When I first came to Switzerland, my job was right up my alley. I could play to my strengths. I was doing analysis work on what companies were doing in the insurance industry and how they were handling different products. I had to cover a lot of material and it was self-focused work. I presented my work directly back to my employer so I established a good relationship there. I didn't have to worry about any intervening supervisors. I knew this would be a good arrangement for me to get my start on the new phase of my career and it was.

Next, I worked in an event management organization. I was doing business development but events were what you did to develop the business. It was an entire climate change. I brought people from all across the world together to think up new ideas and then develop their business side. I worked with the business people to figure out what they needed – to build a new product or to solve a problem. I had to sort out the questions they wanted answered. My role was to take away the information and figure out the puzzle. When I had some answers, we brought all of those people together again and started to make the new challenge happen. That big job shift got my thinking going. I really enjoyed it.

Right now, I'm basically doing a communications role. I've always been fascinated by the challenges of communicating effectively. When I was younger, I had to work on that a lot. In the firm where I work now the concept of thought leadership is their bread and butter. The idea is that thought leadership and learning groups make the difference in market position. I work for the director who works for the head of finance. I make sure that all communications that go to the client are creative, intuitive and bring out the thought leadership of the group. I'm facilitating events and working with the clients. My input is more creative than on a technical level. In the future I may have to decide if I want a more technical role or if I want to stay with the more creative side. But who knows?

Where does that take me in my career? It's always going to be back down to taking in tons of information and pulling it together. That's what I do best. I started with a self-focused kind of job and then moved further and further away from that until now I am working with a whole variety of people. I think my work is more organizational than when I started. I love assembling a team where everybody uses their strengths. The challenge of the job is all about finding the best fit for the client. Who do we need to bring in to get the best result? I've always got multiple factors going on in my head and I love that. Where can the project go? How can it work? Answering those questions intuitively and creatively is one of those things I really enjoy doing. In a sense it's what I have been doing in my own life for a long time.

Skills I Bring to my Job

I tell people "I have a small dis and a big ability". That's also the advice I give other people about how to describe their disability situation. That's what it's about. You have a gift. Each of us has a gift and it's up to each of us to find it and use it. I have an abundance of energy. I have a mind that grabs things in a practical sense. I see pictures with ideas not just words. Can I figure out a model or system? Yes. Can I retain numbers and quickly reference them? No. Do I have a quick reference memory for any details at all? No. Can I put conversations into my long-term memory? Yes. Can I reflect on those conversations and figure out their impact as we go along? Yes. I also have a sensitivity (or you might say a hypersensitivity) to the environment. What makes that useful in my job is that I also have the analytical skills and strategies that I can use to manage the environment.

I work in an accounting consulting firm where you can find a whole range of skills. This firm does the audit of various companies. That's quite a stable part of the business and requires a specific technical skill set. Auditors go through the books and make sure that they are sequential and running with the correct processes. A very structured organizationally driven skill set is required for that. Then you've also got all sorts of other business factors causing chaos. That's where I come in. I feel like the client in some ways when I get an account. I have to work with about five or six different people. I pick their brains to find their ideas, assemble them, and then fit them to the needs of the problem.

Looking back, I see that there's consistency in that way of operating. This is what I can do. I realize that all of the chaos and all of the things that I might have done or messed up over the years are actually a gift. I can look at the chaos and start to sort it out, not panic. High stress, high pressure, I can deal. In a pressure situation or an emergency, I'm not thrown off. My body automatically slows down. I think things through and then I react. If a bear comes to your tent or an oxygen mask comes down in your plane, I'm a good person to have at your side. I know this because these things have happened to me. The same thing goes for a work situation.

I am often called on to do presentations. I always feel the pressure of making a presentation especially because I know there will be good speakers participating with me. When I know I have a big presentation coming up, I do lots of preparation. I might start to worry but that's a normal psychological response. I find the pressure helps me focus. I stay alert and do my best. I started practicing this at university and I am really glad I took all of those opportunities to make presentations. It has really paid off. (All students should do this every chance they get.)

I work hard so that I can be recognized for my skills and the things I have done well. I can't just be social and play for the short term like many people do. I play for the long term. It gets me further ahead. I've still got a strong sense of competition but that competitiveness just pulls me forward. It's not why I do things anymore. Do I compete when I do things like running? Yes, but it is a fun competition not what runs my life.

Is my career advancing as fast as I would like? I don't know. There are moments when I think yes and there are moments when I'd say no. Where I work everything is done on a project basis. When your project is completed you go back to the personnel pool to offer your skills and compete for a new spot. So far, I have always had multiple offers and the change is good for me. It keeps me sharp.

How You Find and Develop New Skills

Going forward in my career I've learned that you have to play different roles and develop different skills depending on your situation. I enjoy the changes and the challenges. Where I work now, I'm part of a team all the time. You have to adapt and find ways to work with your team and your project. Just recently, I found out that my team won an award for developing a newsletter. It's an interesting story from the perspective of teamwork and facing challenges in new situations. Two and a half years ago, I started on this new project. The issue was that the client wasn't getting proper thought leadership and market share. In this account we found that we had quite a lot of technical people who were actually getting good feedback when they worked with a client, but they weren't bringing the message of all this great work out to people within the firm, or to people who might be interested in buying the service.

I asked myself "What other examples of this process do we have?" I talked to other people all around the world about the issues and problems they were having in the areas where this firm worked. We gathered examples of the good work and got information about other solutions and pulled it altogether with our success stories in a very basic newsletter format. People thought it was nice but nothing big.

At random, I just happened to meet a creative designer when I was working on another account. She had great images and booklets for her employer. I asked how she did it. She told me there was marketing software that you can use to develop brochures and professional design products. I asked if I could come and sit with her and watch her work. I went for half a day and watched her. I realized that it was really like advanced power point and I knew I could do that. She went on to give me a technical course in the really fancy stuff.

That one-to-one tutorial was exactly what I needed. While we sat together, I explained what I was trying to do. We started searching through the brand name imagery that we had used before on the account. In the end we pulled together this creative design for our newsletter. In two years, we went from having five people who wanted to see the newsletter on a regular basis to one thousand and fifty people. Funny thing, that many people have clicked yes on their computer, to follow our thoughts on leadership. Now it's an award-winning success and it's the success of everybody. It has really helped us strengthen our position in the marketplace.

Another example would be when I worked on a learning and development project. I was invited to sit in with the board of directors at a strategic planning meeting for a presentation to the owners of the firm. I was part of a team with about six or seven partners who were senior managers and then there was me. They were all two or three levels ahead of me in the organizational chart but I was in charge of putting together a learning map for the company.

How did I land there? The team leader for that board meeting was the partner I had been working with in risk management. That division is basically a lot of incredibly intelligent people who do mathematical modeling along with a lot of other people just really going mad all the time with new ideas to sell business. The focus was just to sell business. We didn't really stop and think or try to be very logical. I proposed that we bring in another partner who came from the accounting side of the firm. He had the very logical, sequential, processing that you might expect from someone trained in accounting. We got him in as my partner and our official learning leader. My role was to brief him. I was studying mass amounts of paper and feeding the information to him. I surveyed the learning programs. I think I was reading two and a half thousand pages every week. I sent back to him my analysis of the key issues with the courses, the key themes and programs. This is one of the other little things that I found out that I do well. I can take lots of information and make it simple. That was why the team leader wanted me at the meeting.

The purpose of this big discussion was to decide on the strategy that should be adopted in the learning and development division to make their presentation to the company's executive board. I sat in those group meetings and I didn't do anything for two and a half days. A couple of the other partners actually asked the boss why I was there. The boss just said to me, "You are here because I know you're going to come up with something for us." Of course, I knew what the others didn't seem to see their way past. You can't present fifteen pages of information, one after the other, on every course we were proposing to the board. You had to have an overall picture of our plan. About five minutes later, the visual came to me. I drew the learning map and turned to my boss and said "What we're doing looks like this?" He just stopped the meeting. He showed them the visual plan and said, "This is our curriculum guys. Now we just put the courses in the different parts of the training outline."

Designing the learning map was really exciting and it was really kind of funny from my side. What that group of senior partners needed was somebody to actually paint the picture for them. Our team needed a visual of what we were actually trying to do and seeing pictures is what I do. After that we needed accountants and people with very strong organizational and structuring skills to actually write the technical framework for what the courses should do. Then we could have a discussion across fifteen courses about how to build up those skills. Finally, we met with people who are more detail oriented to finish it up. There it was: a team success. They still use that template across the organization today.

What you learn about yourself

I don't think of myself as learning disabled anymore. I wouldn't use the term now. Calling it a learning disability is a way of labelling a reaction or a series of emotions that I experienced. It's just a label that describes what things were like when those behaviours and reactions were unconscious and affecting me without me being aware of their effect. The fact is that over time these behaviours and reactions have become conscious and I've developed ways to look after them. Now I unconsciously look after them and work around them.

Do I declare a disability at work? No, at the office I don't think you should automatically. You need to think it through. Business being what it is, I don't think everyone has your best interest at heart. In general, business claims to be striving for diversity but in reality, they are striving for profit. I see businesses supporting lovely causes as long as it's no trouble and the lip service is good for business. In the end it's the numbers and the delivery that counts to them.

You need to be your own self advocate, to fend for yourself and tell people what you need and why it's important. It's up to you to be responsible for yourself. One of the biggest challenges I see in the various firms I work with all across different countries is to get people to actually look after themselves. With all the energy I have, it's a necessity for me to go and do the things I need to be at my best. I can't just go along and expect everything I need to be done for me automatically. If I don't take action or speak up things won't work out.

How much you want to discuss your work style as a disability often depends on your boss. My first boss after I moved to Switzerland "got it." I asked him if having a disability would affect my job with the company and he said not as long as I did my work. Then he told me people suspected he had Asperger's and he wanted to know where he could go to get tested. We had a laugh and that was it. With him, we would get a project and I would arrive at six in the morning and we would work until six at night. We would do that for two or three days. With that level of intensity we could really get things done. Then he would send me home to get a break. He said he needed one too. It was a good partnership. He used to say that working with me was like working with his son but it may not always turn out that way.

My current boss is a female director. She is my second or third female boss. She is very career oriented, exceptionally sharp and brilliant. She is articulate and very supportive but some of her comments are a bit abrupt. Sometimes I have to deflect that because I know it's not what's in her heart. Her style is rough, which is fine because sometimes I need that and I'm not going to say I don't. The difficulty is that the communication is indirect. She tells you what you need to do but you've got to figure out what the real meaning is. You need to decode the instructions. This is harder for me. It reminds me of searching for ways to work with some of the professors I had at university.

The company I work for is set up on a project basis. You often get a new supervisor with your new project. I like the variety but I have discovered that one of the most influential things for me is who I work for. It can be tricky to adapt. I've worked for two or three really different, but great bosses. My first boss was incredibly bright and intelligent. He picked things up really quickly and he was very personable. He was team oriented and social. He would take people out for lunches, dinners, team events. He really paid attention to getting the best out of people for delivery to the client.

I actually did the hiring interviewing for another person I worked for. He was my recommendation because his style was open, direct, to the point and challenging. He also had this other side that was incredibly generous and warm-hearted. This boss would tell me straight to the point what he wanted to do and how he wanted to do it. He would see the simplest way through. We were a powerful team because he knew he couldn't analyze masses of information the way I could. He would say, "Get that fourteen hundred pages down to ten and I'll make it really perfect. You get the key points out, and I'll finesse it because that's what I do best."

I loved his challenges too and his style in doing it. He would tell me what to do with a reason behind it. If he felt something wasn't done right, he would explain why. It was always done so I could crisply and clearly see the problem and what was required. It was done by getting to the point on the issue, not on the person. He wasn't trying to take me apart. That was the brilliance about him. You could get on with the project and get it right. We had really competing styles but the way we managed it they were opposite styles that worked well together. We were a great pair. He always did the personal aspect with business too. I felt we treated each other like family and that is quite unusual in the business culture. It was never just business, business, business. There was always that full element to accomplishing things.
Given my working style probably all of these changes are a good thing for me. The novelty keeps me sharp and motivated to succeed.

Family Life

Raising my kids makes me feel like I'm moving on to the next phase of my life. In university it was you all by yourself. You absorbed the information. Then you fed it back in an exam or paper. That was the whole deal. Now it's not just me and I have to balance work and family life.

My wife is brilliant. She is a linguist and she works as a translator. I love her to death. Our children are six and four. We had lots of time with my daughter. We had almost two years in advance of my son's arrival. I spent a lot of time with her as she was developing. Now she's fantastic. Sure maybe she has a temper tantrum but only once in a while. My son hasn't had as much time with us as his sister has. It was not because of not wanting to have time alone with him but obviously because of more demands. He's also a different child. He has his own personality and he's like his dad. My daughter likes to read books, talk and play games. She is already trilingual and set on a positive path. My son is very motor-oriented. He plays with his train set building things and constructing things outside if possible. He is naturally into sports and that's what he loves. He is on his bike every single day. He rides with me to the daycare and back on his own bike even though he is only four. He is always moving and always wants to be outside.

I have an interesting job and I enjoy it. I may have had a great day at work but when I come home to the kids, who cares? The children can take and they can give but both my wife and I need to use a ton of energy to look after them. There isn't family around to give us a break or help us balance the work load. We do have good friends across the road. They look after the kids for an hour or two. We do the same for them. We've got a little empty lot beside us and a quiet street where all the kids run around and play. The more kids, the more fun they have and the more parents can just chill out and have a coffee and watch them. It only takes two or three hours to sit and have coffee and relax to make a very big difference. If we don't recharge it's disastrous.

It is really important to make sure you spend enough time with your partner. We both believe this but unfortunately, in terms of a priority, it tends to get sidelined. Communication with my wife is extremely important and I know I don't invest enough in it. Even though I know I should, I still don't find more time. But she knows where my heart is and she knows she can trust that. We share the view that right now the really important goal is caring for our children.

I can stand here with my hand on my heart and say "My children are my number one priority. My wife and my family come first." But I have to take time for myself. All of the stuff you talk about beforehand about what's involved in getting married or having children is important, but really for me in the day to day what I needed to talk about was being selfish. I do a lot of bike riding and cycling and running. If I don't do that, I don't cope and I don't recover. I've had quite a few times where I've burnt myself out. I've been just kind of sick and knocked out for two or three days. I was physically exhausted and mentally wiped out. You have all these competing priorities. You've got to go to work. You've got to manage your energy at work. You come home and young children are exhausting. They don't sleep through the night. They disturb you in a million ways. You need time with your wife. But I need to keep my fitness routines to balance myself out. If you neglect yourself it all falls apart. That's what I mean about being selfish.

Managing the day-to-day

Figuring out what I can do and what I can't is the trick of getting through the day. I absolutely have to manage my energy. For me it's all about mixing and matching my energy levels to the situation. On the plus side I can go with more energy longer and harder than almost anyone. But I have had to learn to be selfish and not just at home. When I say being selfish, I mean it's saying "I really need this now." For example, if my boss wants an early morning meeting tomorrow, I will say, "No. I'm going for a run. It's important. If you want me to be optimal all day tomorrow, the run is the best idea. I'll be in at nine." The boss says okay and it works out.

I do my best actual learning and retention in the morning. That hasn't changed since I was in school. I always went to morning courses if I could. I have a two and a half hour block of serious work time at the start of the day. Then it's odds and ends jobs before lunch. That's the stuff that doesn't require full attention. At lunch I run and have a little food to re-energize. I give up a little bit of my networking time at lunch but it does mean that I balance myself and that pays off in doing my work well. I'll have a good piece of time to do work after the run and I do really focused stuff. I finish up with odds and ends jobs again and then get in my serious fitness workout. When I go home, I can have quality time with the kids.

My wife knows she can count on me to pick up the children on the way home or do the morning routine. We do whatever works best for the day's schedule. I may have to go to the store for groceries. I'll have a list with ten things and I'll get you five, three, or maybe two. I've got to take a written list and even then, who knows what you're getting. I do the cooking now. It's surprising but true! I have to because nobody else knows whatever the heck to do with what I bring back from the store. I make it up as I go along and hope it comes out alright. At the end, I get a nice thing to eat or I get a real mess. I enjoy the cooking and nobody else seems too bothered.

When the children come home, they're allowed to watch a couple of kid's shows like Shaun the Sheep or Tom and Jerry because my wife and I need some time to get dinner ready. There's no other way that we can actually put food on the table. After dinner and putting the kids to bed, I usually have some finishing off from work to do. I'm learning German so I try to do some work on that too. I'm always on a kind of roller coaster the entire time.

Maybe that was a model day that I've just described. In reality, I have to be very flexible. Part of what I like about my work is that it's different every day. I have to travel. I take on different projects. Circumstances change and I like that. It's stimulating. For example, I've had a very long week. I made presentations to seventy-five people. That took a lot out of me as far as energy, nerves, preparation and dealing with everybody there. I always have to keep enough of the good structure in my day to keep myself balanced so that I can function and not crash.

Sometimes I have to finish off priority things at home after the kids are in bed. If I have to work late at night it really disturbs me. By late at night I mean 8:30 until 10 or 11. That's as late as it can get for me. One of the other challenges is that my sleep schedule is being programmed by the kids. A late night or an interrupted night means that I don't sleep very well. If I have a really rough sleep it is okay for one or two nights, but again that's back to throwing off the energy balance and that is not good. I've seen what happens if I don't keep to my fitness routines. I come home frustrated and tired and short-tempered with the kids. I've done that before and I'm not going to repeat it. I don't want my kids to learn from seeing their dad like that. I don't want them to think that it is okay to behave badly if you are tired or frustrated. If it's a really bad day, my wife will just say "Time to go on your bike" and vice versa. I do the same for her. For me now the bike is like the chill out room that I learned to use in school. It's all about energy management at home and at work. I have to put that first and I have to work with my spouse on this.

How I Learned to Manage my Energy and my Learning Style

Probably I learned five to ten per cent of what I needed to know over the last ten years. Sixty-five or seventy per cent I learned at university and twenty-five per cent in high school. Let's put it this way. It was at high school that I realized that I was okay. I saw that I did some things very well and some things really poorly. I realized that it was actually myself plus the environment that I needed to control to do my best. What ended up happening in high school was that I became aware. What was unconscious became conscious. I saw there were things I could do to make a good outcome.

In university, managing was still a conscious effort. There were some challenging situations but it was alright to be challenged then. I know it was a pain at the time but I was actually happy later that I knew how to react in those kinds of frustrating and stressful situations. It was basically a good environment for me there and I had people to help me. I needed to be highly focused on sorting things out and trying to do those things that worked for me. I was consciously working at setting my environment and my routines so that I could do my school work.

Here's an example. After a few weeks of classes I realized that I had to deal with my distractibility. I wasn't getting things done. I looked at my room and decided there was too much stuff in it. I couldn't focus. I decided that to work well I needed to clear my room and get rid of all the clutter and distractions. I put the desk facing the wall and closed the window. Some parents might think that kind of situation isn't right for a student but it was just what I needed. This was the kind of thing I had to sort out.

Where I work is still important to me. My distractibility is still there but by now it is my subconscious bias to choose an environment that works for me. At work they moved me to a desk area with six other people. Right away, I found myself a private work booth. When I need to do high focus projects I try to work from home. I automatically know what I need to control in my environment and I find a way to do it.

I think it's important for children to learn that sort of thing at as young an age as possible. You want them to automatically use the right strategy. They may not actually realize what or why they are doing it until they reflect on it later. This is where feedback comes in. It's really helpful if someone can go over these strategies with you. Even though the situations may seem different on the surface, children can learn to see the patterns and how to manage. The big challenge is to get children to train themselves so that their conscious decision is a good one and not one that gets them into trouble. Then later it becomes unconscious and easy. The sooner this happens, the better it is for everyone.

I learned a lot from rowing. I loved rowing. It was about tempo and peace and tranquility. Besides being a healthy choice to be active, I think the thing that any sport does is teach you responsibility for yourself. That's a skill that we all need. It also helps you figure out how to deal with other people. In rowing you have to be there. You have a place and you've got a team of people who need you to be there. You probably find that you get better with practice and that's an important lesson to learn. Who knows how well you can do? At the very least you are going to have fun and you're going to learn a sport.

Eventually, I learned how to take care of my body. You learn that diet is important. If you've been away from a healthy diet for a stretch you start to notice. Sugar gives you nothing by way of nutrition and the energy doesn't last. I've also learned that if you read the label on foods at the store and the list of ingredients is bigger than your finger, you probably don't want to eat it. Even at university, I always tried to eat a healthy diet. I've always had a big reaction to that additive stuff. I want to eat fresh and healthy foods. It makes a big difference to me and the way I function.

I know that many people use caffeine and alcohol and smoking to manage their stress and energy levels. I've learned that the effect of those substances for me is not what you might expect. My reaction to alcohol is very interesting. I like wine and I like the flavors of beer but more of any of it doesn't make me any happier. It doesn't actually do anything for me so why put a bunch of this stuff in my system? The most that will happen is that I will feel sick the next day.

Smoking and drinking alcohol are two things that somebody with a learning disability might like to stay away from. Most of the people I knew with a learning disability at university didn't drink. We had enough trouble controlling ourselves without adding in alcohol or drugs. Look at how many people with Attention Deficit Disorder (ADD) end up in prison. I guess they say about a third of the prison population has ADD. You wonder if the ones who get to university are the ones that don't drink or use drugs. As for smoking, it still makes me sick and it doesn't have a very good long-term health record either.

Caffeine is something that I can use to manage my energy but I have to use it with caution. Those highly caffeinated energy drinks don't do me any good. Red Bull makes me sick if I even smell it. The funny thing is I love coffee. I make my own in a little Italian cappuccino maker. It's a nice process to go through and I can use it as a treat in stressful times. I have to make a calculated decision about whether to have a coffee or not. It's a two cup maximum per day and I can't have coffee after five o'clock or I just physically won't go to sleep. If I feel my sugars are low, I might have an iced tea or a coke. I can use those things as a refresher.

We all do like rewards for ourselves. One of the key ways that I keep motivated and making good decisions is rewards. The challenge is finding the right rewards. Now it's sometimes having a nice coffee or doing something with the children. I get a thrill out of watching them play with a new toy or go skating or learn a new skill. Going for an extra-long bike ride or going to a different mountain and seeing new scenery is great. It doesn't have to be material stuff to be a reward. Sometimes it's the small little things like stopping and taking a pause and realizing that you've done something well. If you don't do that it's bad for you. I've known this for a long time.

The thing is I have to be flexible and aware in managing my energy. Every day I have to use all of those techniques and make all of those decisions, conscious and unconscious, to keep the balance in my life. If you use the bell curve to describe my energy cycles, this is what happens, statistically speaking. When I was younger there was always the volatility on each side of the curve. I was always sliding from one side to the other and going to the extremes. High-low! High-low! I know now that I don't want to hit the 97th percentile. It's bad! It's better to just bounce around the middle of the curve and recognize when you are heading to either end. If you soar to the top, then you fall down. Oh, it happens once or twice and then it's happening over and over again. It may seem good at points but eventually you realize that before you go all the way up to the 97th percentile you had better get out. Woah! Slow down and take a break because the next stop is going down. When that happens you need to get some support. Recover and sleep. Over time you come to figure out how to inhabit the more normal area of the bell curve. Most of the time you are balancing in the middle zone and that is much easier to manage.

How Things Change

It's funny but now when I am studying to learn German, I find that I trust myself and my intuition to guide my learning in a way that I didn't when I was younger. I couldn't tell you why, but I just started believing in myself. Now I realize I'm never going to sit down and just learn the language. What I need to do is figure out the system and structure of the language. Communicating the whole idea is the point for me not necessarily the finer details. The corrections I need are about what is systemically wrong. What differs from before is that I have confidence to follow my unconscious guess. I have found that 80 per cent of the time it's right. My self-confidence is still a battleground for me but I don't beat myself up as much anymore. I have more fun learning new things and I get more retention.

As you get older, your responsibilities and pressures change. At university and before, you have only your school to worry about. You might get stressed over writing exams or handing in assignments but you can go and do your sport. You relax and you get yourself some food. When you are older you realize it's not that easy. There are many important things in your life. In my specific situation, I have work with high stress. Sometimes I need to travel. I've got jobs to do for the family and the house. I've got the marketing to do and cooking. I have my wife and children to spend time with and support. I've got rent and the necessities to provide. There are all these things in my life now to think about and that need my attention.

When you're a kid you think you've got lots of time but you don't actually get that later on in life. You have all these other pressures and all of these other fun things that you want to do but you've only got the same amount of time to get it all done. "I'll do it tomorrow!" doesn't work anymore. Now I have to ask myself those basic questions about balancing time and energy and get focused quicker. My biggest challenge since growing up is being more physically and mentally exhausted.

As I get older, I have to be more selfish. I know this probably doesn't sound right, but I have to be sure to take care of myself. If I don't manage my energy nothing goes well. You still have your patience tried, over and over again in many different ways and you still have to use the same coping skills. I'm very sensitive to the times when I'm not doing what I should be doing in dealing with my family. I don't want to be a poor example for my kids. I find this can happen when I'm stressed from work and I'm more tired. I try to catch myself before I go too far.

The things I worry about now seem different. Maybe it's going through a tough job situation or supporting my family that concerns me. You have your family, your peers, your friends and your career to consider. Perhaps you have to make a really challenging decision that affects not just you but family and friends as well. These may appear to be bigger issues, but I think the things I worry about today come back to the same very basic questions I had to ask myself at university: Where do you put your time and energy? How do you keep your balance? If I found the answers to those questions and learned how to handle those life experiences, I know I can do it now.

Success and self-confidence do change things. After a certain amount of years, you build up some financial stability as well as experience. That's actually very helpful. You don't have student loans. You don't always have to be worried about your income or supporting your family. You get some sort of foundation laid. After all of those years of work I have put a base down. There are other things that I want to work for but now I've got some flexibility in my life. Which means you can think, "Oh, I'm actually okay."

Some Things don't Change

I know that I still have the same challenges related to my learning disability. I have issues with memory and I still have work to do on listening. My attention span cuts out my listening. My mind always jumps around when I can see a parallel situation. I still have to read things over a few times and I still have to be able to control my environment to focus for work or study. I get those intense focuses where I lock on and don't do anything else until I burn myself out. I could read all day. At work it depends on the material I need to cover. If I read an action book or some kind of story that really catches my imagination, I might read all night or at least until my wife comes in and turns out the light.

I am aware of a whole lot of the things that are going on around me all at once. Even while we are having this conversation, I'm thinking about eight other things and noticing the sounds and all the action. I guess you could say I am extra sensitive to my environment. I have to work to focus on the important thing at hand. I find this extra sensitivity is there in a social sense too. The impact I have on somebody else is very important to me. I feel the pain of a misstep. It's a hyper-sensitivity really. Rather than being helpful sometimes that sensitivity can work the other way.

What is important to me on a personal level is figuring out how I can help other people. I manage to do some coaching and mentoring at work and I enjoy that. I seem to have about four or five people who use me as an informal coach/counsellor. I just give them frank feedback and I encourage them to do better. One of my happiest moments was helping a colleague get a promotion. It was the right job for that person and both of us felt we had accomplished a good thing for the group and the success of our project.

When I'm at work, I find that I can sometimes get really mad and frustrated if people aren't paying attention to personal things, like saying thank you and remembering who you are. I'm not the best with names, but I'll remember a face and at least make an effort to remember a name. I'll say my thanks and express my appreciation. I've managed teams, and I know that when you push your team, you also have to reward them with a lunch or doing something nice for them. I always want to make sure that I treat people well, like humans should. I think that's a belief and a skill set that my dad ingrained in me from day one. There were times when I wasn't treated so well and I think that helps you to have the sensitivity to say I'm not going to do that.

I'm still a frustrated person. I am offended by rules that don't work very well or don't work for everyone. I also get frustrated if I make a spelling mistake. Or if something doesn't work perfectly. I think I'm overly sensitive if somebody spots an error of mine especially in my publishing. I know it's natural to have frustration. I just have to let the things that frustrate me go because I can't make many of them any different. I say that things are frustrating, but it's more my impatience. I'm not really a frustrated person in a fundamental sense. I'd love to spend more time on my bike. I want to spend more time with my kids. I don't want to work as much but then work is interesting and fun. After I spend the weekend with the kids, I'm exhausted and I want to go back to work. I also need time to slow down. I want all of the above and I try to keep it all in balance. That's why I should say that I have moments of frustration. Really what I always want is to improve and make things better.

What is the perfect world really? The kids go to daycare but I would love to take some more time with them the way my wife does. If I take more time with them, then we have to give up some income. That means we can't have the same lifestyle. Maybe we can't go to Canada to see my parents or we can't go as often to see my wife's parents. It means we lose that special time. I'm still searching and I'm still frustrated trying to do it all. But the benefit of a more complicated life is that you have the whole positive side of things to enjoy. It's all part of life.

Learning at Home and School

You hope that you are laying a positive foundation for your kids in your daily life together. How much influence do I have? How much does my wife have? It's interesting to ask these questions because I think that modeling can be a positive or a negative factor. Children see the way you treat them and the way you deal with other people. You talk to them about how to handle problems. But I'm not perfect. I have yelled. I have screamed. I've lost my cool, but I think everybody does. My friends, who don't have ADHD, have the same problems as I do with their kids. They tell me about their little ones not listening, breaking things or ignoring them when they try to stop them from doing things that are dangerous. Everybody has those problems. Everybody has reacted in ways like me. But on the plus side, I'm quick to catch myself and get off for a walk. I tell them, "Dad needs to go. I'll be back and we'll talk." Having a sort of calmness around them allows people to interact with their children properly. I try to model that too.

Since we are living in a German-speaking environment, I've started studying German at home in the evenings. There is no other time available. It can be a bit of a challenge to get refocussed but as I mentioned earlier it's interesting learning a new language now. There are times when I'm studying and I'm useless at it and I feel terrible. My children are now passing me. That gives me a big push to get going. I say I'm learning German for the kids but it's also for me because it's going to mean more career opportunities so I have lots of motivation to refocus at night. It's important to find your motivation. You have to ask yourself, why is it worth the effort? Finding the answer makes it easier to achieve your goals. That's a big lesson I want to stress with my kids.

One of the other lessons I am teaching my children is to question things. It's important for them to learn to trust their intuition and ask even though it might cause a problem at first. This got my daughter in trouble at swimming class. She could basically jump into the shallow end of the water and paddle around and support herself. For the safety of the class the teacher wanted to have water wings on everybody. The teacher made all the kids, even though some of them could actually swim, have water wings. My daughter was upset. I said to her, did you ask why? She hadn't. So, I said, ask the teacher why. When she asked, the teacher's response was, "It's important. You need to wear them." There was no discussion or explanation. My response was, "Next time when she gives you that response just jump in to show her that you can swim." Next time that's what my daughter did.

When I came to pick her up that day, the teacher said she had disobeyed her. My daughter had jumped in without the water wings. I said "Good for her. She did that to show you that she could swim." Then we had a discussion. I asked her if she ever explained why she had that rule. I told her that I fully supported her concern for the safety of the class and I understood that water wings made it easier for her to watch. Then I asked her if she ever thought to say to a couple of those kids, "Yes, we need to do this but why don't you just jump in quickly and show me what you can do. Then we'll put the water wings on after and that will be our deal." The teacher actually looked at me surprised.

I also said to the teacher, "By the way I want her to challenge you and if it's inappropriate, tell me and I'll have a word. I'm there to support you. I respect you and I don't want my children to disrespect you. I just want my daughter and my son to speak up. I want them to know that they can think themselves through a problem and that they shouldn't just accept a situation that doesn't seem right." We'll see how it goes.

I've learned a lot of things just watching how children play. I've noticed children with attention problems. I've seen how they react and how they lash out. I see the tension and the way they look socially unfit. It makes me think of my younger self. This is how children can seem if you actually do not realize that their behaviour may mean something else. It's a call that they're bored. They want friends. They want to be stimulated. Their brains are very intelligent and they need something to take their attention. Fundamentally the child needs to be active. I see this. My children's behavior does change when they are bored. I don't want to say that my children have ADD but they do need to be engaged. Kids are very social. They are very sensitive to other people's reactions to them. They need to be having fun. They need to be challenged. They need to be doing things that are positive and that give them a sense of accomplishment.

One of my big passions in life is exploring how to start teaching younger children some of the skills that I didn't learn or really develop until university. How can this happen in the early grades? When I think about the frustrations people have about the school systems, what I see are the teachers worrying about the school and the class versus the individual. Someone with ADHD (Attention Deficit Hyperactive Disorder) needs the investment of time and attention especially when they are young. The time to get those coping skills is as soon as possible. When kids are in high school at fifteen or sixteen with all the chemicals and emotions going through their heads, they aren't really receptive to talking about coping skills. I'm not sure how but I hope you can build the foundation for success when a child is young. That's what we are trying to do with our children.

I've got two unique, beautiful children. I want the best for them. I hope we can give them the kind of experiences that will put them on a positive path for life. In our city there is a school that has programs for sports, music, art or dance. It takes the students one extra year to graduate. I think that school has the right way of doing things. It allows the students to get their education and develop their passion whatever it is. If they go full tilt into sports and they're superb, that's great, but they will always have an education. They will learn to have balance in their life and that is very important.

I'm putting away money to create an education fund for my children. I hope they will go overseas to school when they are older. I think that was one of the best things that I did. I went away to experience a different culture and to experience how different people operate. It's interesting and you learn to understand that difference is okay. You also have to stand up for yourself. It may all be new and you may have no money but you have to figure out what the heck to do. Standing on your own two feet and knowing you can is really important. That's what I want for them.

Sharing the Secrets

I try to help people out by using my own story. How did I deal with myself and all that comes with having a disability? I like to help kids and mentor people or students who are going through similar situations to mine. Mentoring and coaching is for all ages and not just for work.

The education system dealing with the child is one thing but I think what is really missing is parent coaching. There are a lot of parents who have children with ADD who need coaching to actually understand their children. If parents know what their child is experiencing, it helps them deal with what they are doing at home. I think it would be a big help to the parents to actually talk to somebody who can say "Do you know that your child is not a bad child? Your child is not doing this to piss you off." Kids with a learning disability may run away. They will vent their frustration in ways that are not very beneficial, but it will be a lesson for them if you help them deal with the poor choices they have made. Eventually the kids will discover a better way. It would really help if parents could understand that.

Parents play an absolutely huge role in the child's development. They always do and they always will. My father is still who I would go to for counsel. In my family we are all convinced my dad and I are both learning disabled. He still forgets things and he can't handle the grocery lists any better than me. He has to manage his diet and take good care of himself. Both he and my mother are doing pretty well. Of course, they have the health thing here and there that holds them up from time to time. My dad is still a bundle of energy. He is still working as a consultant. He says he needs to keep his brain going. That is the one thing that is the essence of people with ADD. Intellectually, they have to keep themselves challenged all the time. I'm the same.

With a couple of my neighbours we discuss parenting. I think I can help those younger families see the unconscious ways they are operating and how they could consciously change things to make them go more smoothly. For example, after I talked to my friend about his child, I saw that the child needed a place where he could calm down and cool off. I suggested that the guy should look for a place where his child could have a space of his own. He cleared out his study and now his son goes there to be alone and think. That study is the child's comfort zone now and nothing goes badly in there for him. My friend said, "This really helps and I can go somewhere else and work". I don't think he understood yet but it was enough for him that it worked.

This dad is also out there for about two hours every morning with his son riding his bike and doing some fitness things to try and tire him out for kindergarten. Something's wrong and something is wrong with what happens at the kindergarten. That child needs to run and be active so he can get some peace. The boy is a hilarious kid. He is bright and he touches your heart. He comes screaming down the hill on his bike. He is crazy on that bike but it's totally controlled. He has acquired skills on a bike that really wowed all of us. He likes hockey too and sports of all kinds. That is his out. It helps him get himself balanced and find that sort of quietness so he can absorb new things. His dad is with him, teaching him a coping skill.

I love to see all of this happening but I wonder how long the dad can keep going with all of these activities. The dad says it's great. He is getting in shape himself and losing weight. I advised him to start thinking about community sports and activities for the child. That way the child could learn to balance his energy with groups outside the family. He could try something like organized hockey and soccer teams. Maybe he could take extra classes or some private lessons in something he likes that will build his skills. This way as the child grows, he will get stronger and more skilled. It will just become a natural thing to manage his energy in good ways.

I talk to another couple who are struggling with a child that the school system is trying to peg into a box of some kind. They haven't had any proper psychological assessments. The teacher is saying "Have you thought about medication?" The doctor is saying," I can write you a prescription if you'd like. Have you thought about these other alternatives?" But they're not getting a full picture anywhere. What can medicine really do? What are the pros? What are the cons? Try finding out the long-term psychological costs of Ritalin and other medications. Where are the research studies? There are major medical issues going on here. There have been several articles in the press lately which showed the problems with drug use for children. There's evidence of mental health effects and kids having some major health problems in the longer term. Those studies are getting put away and ignored because of the benefits of the drugs. Am I against drugs? No, I just think their use needs to be well thought out. It should be a conscious decision and unemotional.

Parents get pushed into a situation with their children which is emotional. They are trying to manage their child who is taking all of their energy. They've got work. They've got stress. If they've got other children as well, they've got a whole other set of issues to deal with too. These parents don't have the time to slow themselves down to make what is the best decision for the child. A struggling child's parents are listening to all these professionals and talking to more. They are trying to make these decisions and nobody really knows the whole picture either.

When I see these parents, who are my friends, I feel the pressure and the confusion I remember. I think they are probably going through what I just described. From my own experience I point out some skills that they can work on: when your child reacts wildly you've got to tell him, "No, no, no!" You've got to be strict and firm. At the same time, you've got to show him that you love him. You've got to constantly build his confidence. Since he's young, his confidence is sapped by his struggles and even by stupid things that might not be about his parents. It can be as simple as someone saying something mean that sets things off in the wrong direction.

In my experience kids with learning disabilities are sensitive. They are overly sensitive to everything. If you think about it, their difference gives them two of the most difficult things a young child needs to deal with. One is that painful sensitivity and the other is the need to fit in. Children don't feel accepted if nobody is playing with them. Having friendships and kids to play with is very important in a child's life. When they are frustrated with trying to fit in, children with learning disabilities may withdraw or react either physically or violently and do stupid, impulsive things that turn more kids off. Really inside of them all they want is a friend. It's hard to explain this vicious circle to the kids themselves because it is actually really counter-intuitive. Finding out what's going on in the child's mind is important. The earlier parents can get to understand how their child is thinking, the better it is. It allows parents to offer alternatives and help their child change their destructive behaviours. Explaining what's going on to other parents and their kids can help too.

A teenager with learning disabilities has the added complications of plenty of hormones floating about. The balance or lack of balance of chemicals in your head is a factor that stands out to me. I remember it well. At puberty, as any medical doctor will tell you, there's an explosion of disorientating things running through your body and it's not just you. It's everyone else in the class too. That's the environment the person is in at fourteen and that is why the earlier the parents can get to understand how their children are thinking the better it is. The best you can give a teenager is to keep them safe and offer some sort of stability and confidence. When I say keeping them safe, I mean letting them experience things. Let them fall down but help them get back up. Talk with them about what went wrong and how it might have worked out better. Getting out of those destructive circles is one of the biggest challenges that people like me face.

I vividly remember, from age fourteen onwards, what I was going through. I still have it with me now. I can experience it sitting here and I can tell you what it felt like. I try to make a positive contribution as an adult who has been through it by offering my own experience. I know learning disabilities take a variety of forms and I wonder about other people and how they find their coping skills. This is how it looks to me. I'm not a psychologist. I'm just speaking strictly and practically from my experience.

THE VIEW FROM OUTSIDE

After the evening I spent with John, I came away with a sense of the energy and enthusiasm with which he embraces his busy and successful life. He is clearly enjoying the opportunities his exciting and productive life offers. He has a cautious regard for his accomplishments and seems a bit bemused by how well things have worked out. During our time together, I saw no hint of the effort he must have been expending to control the "eight tracks of information" that still play through his mind. He is a long way from the angry, acting-out teenager of his youth. Those struggles are hard to imagine when you see him now.

John tells us stories of his successes and set-backs. He details for us the complex system of strategies and skills that he uses to maintain a successful business career in a high-powered multinational firm while balancing his responsibilities as a husband and parent. He paints vivid pictures of his daily life at work, at home and in his neighbourhood. He gives us a real sense of the "roller coaster" he lives from day to day and the optimism and determination that have enabled him to excel. He estimates with percentages the timing and impact of various interventions and strategies. He uses the image of the normal curve to illustrate his energy flow variations and the balance he has created in his life. We can see what he means about his professional skill of "communicating in fresh and meaningful ways." He even offered me the notes he had prepared for our conversation. I felt I could understand how highly he must be regarded by his clients and team mates.

Learning to manage himself and his environment allows John to succeed. He has the habit of analyzing his failures and celebrating his successes. His insights into that process help him raise his own children and offer valuable mentoring and coaching to others. Over the years John learned to work with the chaos of his internal world and find ways of expressing his considerable strengths. He mastered the art of seeing his environment in ways that allow him to use his strengths. Now he has made a career of helping other people manage the challenges they face. That ability allows him to confront the business problems of his clients with confidence. He uses his energy and his knack of visualizing and organizing ideas as key assets. He offers a different point of view and practical creative options that he communicates in convincing and innovative ways. Even though John worried about his ability to convey his ideas effectively at university, he has clearly turned communication skills into an area of expertise.

It is important to John to be able to help others break out of the painful cycles that limit their lives. He worked hard to recognize the paths to his own success and he is hopeful that his experiences will offer solutions for others. His descriptions of the inner life of a child with learning disabilities are a powerful reminder of the challenges those early years present. They also give us a window onto John's own childhood struggles. His reflections on his own life reveal how his parents' support and a climate of informed feedback from a variety of sources allowed him to understand his behavior and gain an awareness of better options. He describes the process of moving from being at the mercy of his unconscious negative behaviors to an awareness that allowed him to take control and make better choices. Spotting and understanding the destructive circles of behavior that trapped him was critical to finding his way forward. Now good options are the automatic choice and he feels that he has "a little dis and big ability."

At university, John came to terms with the realities of managing his disability in new and challenging environments. He accepted that his life would not be ordinary so he decided to "go with it and see what he could pull out of his back pocket" to deal with the funny things that result. He developed professional credentials, travelled and sampled other places and cultures. Now he has a career, a house and a family in a multicultural community where he feels at home. He followed his motto of being brave in trying and it has served him well.

John sees his life as complicated but full of good things. Time for career, family and friends are all priorities for him. He still feels the frustrations of his struggles but good options are automatic for him now. He has accepted how critical energy management is to his life and he has put his problems solving skills to work on managing the work and family balance that he values. We are never in doubt about how essential and enabling that balance is. His goal is not to return to the days of rocketing between energy highs and lows. His exercise and nutrition strategies are a stabilizing constant in his days. They are a pleasure for him and they work. When they don't, he rests up, gets support and starts again. He has adopted a practical, business-like approach to keeping all the parts of his complex system in balance and he usually succeeds. Like many people at forty, there are still things that he wants to change but he knows what he has to do to stay healthy in the midst of his busy work and home life. He tells us that his life is not perfect. Yet to an outside observer, it certainly reflects his ability to escape the destructive cycles of behavior that held him back and the many good decision he has made.

8
ALICE WATKINS
University Years

I came to university scared, not really knowing anybody and with the definite sense that I was going to be working against the odds to succeed. I knew I had a learning disability. Dealing with detail is a problem for me, both taking it in and remembering it. I have problems with reading, as well as spelling and grammar and such things that affect my written language. I knew university wasn't going to be easy, but I wanted to be a math teacher so there was no other choice. I had the basic idea that hard work and determination would see me through. What I didn't have was a real understanding of my abilities and the things that I needed to do to accommodate my learning disability at university. The first battle was for me to realize what a person with learning disabilities can achieve. The second was convincing the professors. During my time at university, I came to believe in my ability and understand how to do well. I finally realized that I wasn't stupid. I could make high marks and be one of the top students in the class, if I did the right things and was accommodated in the right way.

My experience at university definitely had its ups and downs. I had two disastrous years and fought my way back from dismissal to the Dean's List for excellence. I think that I have learned from my mistakes and from the things I did right. I hope that others can learn from me and my experiences. I don't want them to make the same mistakes that I did. More importantly, I hope they realize that, even if they do make mistakes, it is not too late to try again. Do not give up just because you have a learning disability. Everybody makes mistakes. Having a learning disability doesn't mean you can't do what you want. It doesn't mean you can't accomplish your dreams.

Getting to University: Against the Odds

I knew I wanted to go to university so I applied to about a dozen places. I didn't think that anyone would take me, so I wasn't going to just try one or two. I felt I was grasping at straws. My average was usually in the fifties or sixties. When the teachers told us that at university we should expect our marks to drop by 20 per cent, I really thought I had no chance of success. Judging from most of my high school years, twenty marks down would have had me failing. Not many students from my school went to university. For a student with a learning disability, the possibility of university or college of any sort seemed an even lower probability. Why bother even applying? What made me any better than the other students from my school who weren't going on? My dream was to become a math teacher and this was the next step. It seemed almost impossible, but I was going to try my hardest anyway.

When I was at high school I mainly looked for just a pass. I think many of my teachers just gave me a pass because of the way I appeared to them. They saw me as very hard working and a nice person, so they gave me a nice little pass. My graduating average turned out to be one of my best averages. It was seventy-five. It was a good average when you compared it to other students. But compared with my previous years, it seemed like a fluke. Maybe these nice teachers wanted to make sure I went on? Maybe they just wanted the school to look good? I didn't know, but I didn't trust that mark. Although I didn't consider what I had done good enough for university, eleven of twelve universities accepted me. That told me something. Somehow I had done well enough to be able to advance to further learning. This is what I had hoped for, but I found it hard to believe that it had really happened.

When I applied to my present university, it was just one of those twelve schools that I was trying. I didn't know anyone at the university, or anyone who wanted to go there. I had no idea if there were people there to help students with learning disabilities. My first visit to the campus was in May of my grade twelve year. My resource teacher told me that there was a transition weekend for students with learning disabilities, so I decided to see what it was like. It wasn't until then that I actually saw the things that had been established in the university to help students with disabilities. I saw that there were people to help and that accommodations were possible. Many teachers in my high school said that I would never get anything like these kinds of adjustments and supports in university. That weekend was very encouraging. I think it was especially important for me to have met some of the staff and some students since I was coming to a university where I knew no one. Not to have any contacts is hard for anyone, but I think it's especially hard for a student with a learning disability. After that weekend I knew this was the university that I wanted to attend and now at least I knew some people there.

First Year: The New and Wild Ways of University

My first year was a scary experience, but it was a learning experience. Coming in, I not only had to adapt to the new and wild ways of the university, but I also had to do a whole lot of extra things to look after my learning disability. I needed to find people as soon as possible to be notetakers. I had to speak about my learning disability to these professors who seemed so authoritative. I had to tell them that I did have a learning disability and then try to work with them to find a good learning situation. Most of the professors that I had my first year tried to a certain extent to help and accommodate me. I think they tried their best, but now I think that the majority of them didn't realize what learning disabilities were, or what my particular learning disability was. It was the first time that I really had to speak out about my learning disability. I didn't know for sure what accommodations I would need at university, or how exactly to explain my situation. It made the year hard, but definitely a learning experience.

I was in a similar situation with the two student tutors who were helping me. I had never had a tutor up to that point, only a resource teacher. It was difficult figuring out how to work with the tutors. One was for economics and the other for psychology. I was trying to learn the basic language for these courses and then trying to help the tutors to understand what my learning disability was. We were all trying to find out what I needed from them. This was hard and to this day I'm still not sure if they really know what a learning disability is. For the most part, they helped as best they could with the knowledge they had.

There were a lot of good things about that first year. My marks were respectable. I made a 61 per cent average. That was pretty much the norm for most of my high school years and well within the range that my high school teachers had talked about for most students. I had passed all five courses and I had learned a lot about myself. I felt that I had a lot better idea about what I could do. I had learned to use my new computer. I had made good contacts with the professors. I had found notetakers. I had made friends and joined clubs. I enjoyed residence life. I had established a routine that worked. I met every week with the counsellor. I carried a notebook to keep me organized and remind me of questions I needed to ask. I was pleased.

I see now that in some senses my first year wasn't the success I thought it was. It's true, I came to a strange environment and I was able to get through. I thought that was the goal. Yet I know now that getting through and being successful are two different things. Somehow that 61 percent average was too much of a security blanket for me. It gave me a booster shot that allowed me to overestimate what I could do. It gave me a false image of what was taking place. In first year, it seemed that almost everything important was covered in class. I know now that hearing the material is a big advantage to me. I didn't need to do a huge amount of independent reading and research to get through. I went to every class and I had notetakers. I talked to the professors. Everyone knew I worked hard and was enthusiastic about my courses. I was always very positive in the way I presented myself. That seemed to be enough.

In some courses I did well and in others I had marks in the fifties. With different study strategies and different exam conditions I could have done much better, especially with those courses in the fifties. I was underestimating my potential in those courses. I have more ability than just getting through. I got those marks without really figuring out how to accommodate for my learning disability.

Year Two: Things Fall Apart

It was a different year. Going into my second year, I was quite confident. I thought that I was ready for bigger and better things. I figured I could take on the world. To protect my career options I was registered in business, so I took the courses required for business. Really I wanted to be a math teacher, so I thought I would take all math and computer courses for my electives. These were the subjects I wanted to teach, so by taking them as electives I would still be headed in the right direction while enrolled in a professional program. I also decided it was best to shy away from English-type courses and English specifically. I was scared of all the reading and the writing assignments. Basically I thought I would go into courses that required very little reading and writing, and used group work and presentations as a method of evaluation. In that way I could accommodate my learning disability. To me it seemed to be a most ideal plan.

Unfortunately, what I had done was set myself up for a fall. When you take so many different courses, there are a lot of differences in the terminology. One word may mean different things, depending on the course you are sitting in. I made charts and visual aids to help me remember the terms and the procedures. I stuck them up all over the place, but I didn't have time to review them. Eventually I didn't have time to make them either. Taped texts weren't available for the math and computer courses, but I didn't think I needed to spend much time reading them anyway. Most of the time was spent on practical work and doing examples. That was good, but I had so much to handle that I couldn't keep up.

Part of the problem was that I had realized that I needed calculus to go on to the education program. I didn't have pre-calculus, but I had taken introductory math in first year. I had done pretty well, so I thought calculus couldn't be that hard. I decided to 'just go for it' and I got departmental permission to try. I soon found out that I had underestimated what was involved in the calculus course.

Another problem was that the network of support that I had set up in my first year was no longer around. Many of my friends had not returned to university. My counsellor went on leave. At the time I didn't see having a different counsellor as a difficulty for me until I tried to work with the new person. I don't believe she really realized what my learning disability was and what I really needed. She didn't feel that I needed all of the time I was requesting from her. She encouraged me to make accommodations directly with the professors and to keep her out of it in a lot of respects. Her approach was to let the professors find a place where I could write exams. In first year my exams could be proctored at the counselling centre. I understand the importance of being independent, but this system did cause problems for me.

For the most part professors were willing to find a place for me, but those places weren't necessarily the best places to stick me and just sticking me somewhere was basically what it was. Sometimes the location would be changed without any notice and the location was often different each time. I did not have a stable place, or necessarily even a quiet place, to be tested. Usually there were a lot of distractions and very little privacy. This was exactly what I was trying to avoid.

Like everyone else, professors are not by any means perfect. They didn't seem to realize how much difference something that seems like a small change to them can make to a student's ability to write a test. For some people, a change in what you expect to take place can have a grave effect. With one of my final exams, the professor told me to meet her at a certain place, at a certain time to write my exam. I was keyed into that and it was a suitable place. I expected to go there and start writing my exam as soon as I arrived. At the last minute, she decided that she didn't want me to write my exam there. It was more convenient for her to move me to a different building. This was not a suitable atmosphere for me to write an exam. It would not have been good for anyone for that matter, because of the level of noise and other distractions. My performance on that exam was terrible.

In another course the professor didn't see that it was helping me to have a special setting to write my tests. He felt I might just as well stay in the classroom. Since I wasn't passing anyway, what was the difference? Why should he take more time to help me find some place to write, even though it might help me be more successful? I failed that course.

Needless to say, although I had started second year with confidence, things did not go too well. To make things even more difficult, over the summer five people who were close to me passed away. One was a close friend and the other four were close relatives. I think that definitely played a part in the difficulties of my second year. I didn't really deal with any of the deaths. I was always doing something else to keep my mind from playing on them. I didn't put enough time into my studies. That year my learning network inside the university broke down, and my supports outside of the university broke down as well. It was a disastrous year. I passed two courses out of five.

When my marks came, the university informed me that I had not met their academic requirements and I would have to sit out for a year. Getting that letter terrified me. I didn't know how I would manage after a year away. As it was, I found it hard to get back into the school routine after even a summer off. I couldn't comprehend what it would be like after sitting out a whole year. I also believed that there were special circumstances contributing to my poor academic performance. The different problems with professors during exams, the breakdown of my network of support both in school and outside. These were all factors that contributed to my poor grades. I also felt that these were all things that could be different if I was allowed to return. I appealed the suspension decision by explaining the grounds for my lack of success. I guess the university accepted this explanation. They let me come back on probation. That told me clearly, "Don't do it again!" I didn't intend to.

During the summer I had to decide whether to choose the math or business program. To me, there was really no decision to be made. It would be math. That was my original goal and that's how I wanted to continue. I transferred out of the business program into the arts mathematics program, so that I could receive credit for all of my business courses. To do this and keep up the program pace, I had to take an extra course. I didn't think it would be a problem. I knew it would be more work, but I thought it would definitely be worth it. I also decided to take a correspondence course over the summer to try to get the calculus credit that I had missed in second year. Calculus was a prerequisite for some of the math courses that I wanted to take. At least that credit would get me a little bit back on track and closer to graduating.

Year Three: A Second Chance

Starting my third year I felt that everything was going to be fine. I saw the previous year as unusually difficult mostly due to circumstances beyond my control. I thought I had developed an excellent plan to get around the problems caused by missing three credits. I was on academic probation. I was carrying an extra course and I still had the correspondence course in calculus from the summer to finish by Christmas. For the majority of the math courses I was taking, I didn't have the prerequisites due to my poor performance in second year. I didn't see the problems. The math department and the Dean's Office had given their permission. I figured the university must think I can do this. If they think I can do it, I must be able to do it.

My counsellor returned and tried to help me pick up the pieces. We tried to understand what had gone on in the year she was away. She recommended a reduced course load. To balance out my program, she advised me to try an English or social science course instead of having so many maths. Rather than avoiding subjects because I was afraid of the reading and written assignments, she suggested I use taped texts to accommodate for my reading problems. I decided to try an English and a psychology course, but I took them along with everything else I needed in math and computers. I thought that was not a bad compromise. It was a little of both and would make us both happy. There was no way I was taking a reduced course load. I wanted to make up for the courses I had lost already.

I think it's important to have people think well of you, and to get advice and support, but it is also important to realize what you really can do. I think a lot of times we don't and I think that can happen to the people helping you too. When it comes down to it, you are the one who makes the choice and has to live with it. You are the one who has to be fair to yourself in estimating your abilities and the task ahead. You can't give up too early, or be too pig-headed either. I think I excel at both of these things, so I guess I can talk from experience. I made my choices that year and they didn't work out very well at all.

By Christmas time I was failing the math and computer courses, but succeeding in the psychology and English course. I was getting marks in the teens and twenties, but I still refused to drop any courses.

I refused to give up, even though to an outside observer it was plain that it wasn't possible for me to pass. This did not help my overall average for the year. It was a tricky situation. I had some personal difficulties again in that first term. My grandmother passed away. Her passing really confronted me with all of the deaths that I hadn't dealt with in the summer following first year. Added to that was the stress of being on probation and having overload courses. I had to write my exam for the correspondence calculus course at Christmas along with all my other exams. The timing couldn't have been worse. Shortly after Christmas I found out that I had failed my calculus course.

You know, I continued on after Christmas. I thought, "I'll do all right. I've only failed a couple of courses. They are half credit courses. I still have enough courses that I can pass. I can still make my three courses and that's enough to get me through." I even tried a supplemental exam for my correspondence calculus course, but it didn't help and it took more time away from my other studies. As the second term went on, I did come into some sense. I was making marks in the teens and twenties in geometry. I did drop that, but by then there wasn't much chance to get too many credits from the year.

When my marks arrived at the end of the year, there was also an official letter telling me I had been dismissed from the university. That really didn't please me. It hit me very hard. Of course, I appealed the decision hoping I could overturn it as I had the previous year. I was able to raise my psychology mark to a credit on appeal, but that still wasn't enough. According to the regulations, I was dismissed.

I made numerous attempts to change my dismissal. I basically became a pen pal of the Dean of Arts. It didn't help. A few days before classes were to begin, I showed up at the doorstep of the Dean's Office. I pleaded with the man to let me in, but he turned me down. I can still hear him saying, "No, there is nothing I can do." This upset me. I knew that I wanted to return some day, so I sought his advice about how to make that possible. He suggested that since English was my highest mark, I might take an English course in my home area. Since I was dismissed, this course would not count as a credit toward my degree. It would help me keep involved with school and build my strength in English. I was still disappointed, but I decided that was what I was going to do.

Before leaving the campus, I had developed a new plan. I decided that taking one English course would definitely not keep me busy enough. No doubt about it, I would go insane with so little happening in my life. My goal was still to be a math teacher. I had not given that up. I decided to see if I could go back to high school and get the pre-calculus that I needed to help me with university calculus. I knew that I needed to take calculus sometime in order to get into an education program. I wasn't going to waste time during this year off. Taking both English and pre-calculus would put the time to really good use. I went back home that evening ready to go back to high school the following morning.

Year Four: A Year Away

Returning to high school was a big challenge. Not necessarily in the sense of taking a step back, but it hit me that I was in classes with the younger brothers and sisters of the students who had graduated with me. I was not in classes with my peers. I was with the friends of my younger brother. This would make school life very interesting.

Everything worked out well at the high school. I arranged to take the English course by correspondence, so that I could attend the classes I wanted at the high school. I took pre-calculus and two additional math classes. I was able to help other students in math. My math teacher arranged for me to teach extra classes to gifted math students from the junior high school. We both thought that this experience would strengthen my chances of qualifying for a teacher education program. I designed and taught a math camp for younger students who were having trouble with the subject. I got excellent marks at high school. It was a pleasant change from the marks I had been receiving at university. It gave me a chance to rebuild my self worth and realize that I wasn't stupid. I was able to have a busy and very successful year there.

Unfortunately, the English course was a different story. I failed the exam and that meant I failed the course. My assignments had been fine, but I had to pass the exam in order to pass the course. I was able to write the exam on my own in a quiet place, but I did not receive extra time to write. My proctor was not allowed to read the questions for me, or read back what I had written so that I could correct it. The exam was disastrous. When I met with the professor to see what could be done about my mark, she showed me my exam. Reading it through many weeks after, I could tell that there were obvious grammatical and spelling mistakes. I believe I could have fixed the majority, if not all of them, with extra time for the proctor to read my answers back to me. As it was, I could tell that the professor's offer of getting a second reader was not going to help my mark. Since the course would not be a credit toward my degree, I decided it wasn't worth the worry. This did not make me feel good, but it meant I didn't need to find a way to write a more satisfactory exam. It seemed best just to move on.

Throughout the year, I had visited and kept in touch with my friends at university. I talked to some of my professors and my counsellor. I made sure they all knew that I was still interested in returning and I kept them up to date on what I was doing. In the spring I made numerous written attempts to get permission to return. The last letter I wrote to the Dean was very frank. I was more straightforward than in my other letters. Normally my personality doesn't lead me to do that. Basically I said: "Look, I've done what you wanted me to do. If there was something else that you wanted me to do, you should have told me. It is my understanding that I have done what you requested and more. I have learned from my experiences in the year off. I should be able to get back to finish what I have started, so that I can move on." Not long after that I got a letter saying that I could return on probation. Finally they had agreed to let me back!

Year Five: Last Chance

It was exciting to get back to university, but it was also very scary. The year back at high school had built up my confidence, but I knew this was my last chance. I decided that I was going to prove to people, including myself, that I could make it at university just as I had in my first year. This time I had the prerequisites for the courses that I had failed before. Now that I had the foundation, the key that had been missing, I was sure that I was well on my way to success in the math courses.

I decided on taking a reduced course load and not so many math courses at once. I selected calculus to capitalize on the recency of my pre-calculus course. I selected an English course, since that had been my highest mark. I tried sociology, since I needed to select another subject area for my degree. I decided to make another change and live off campus. This would take me away from all of the noise and distractions that come with residence life.

At the first set of mid-terms my marks were barely passes. We had tried one way of accommodation and I realized it still didn't work. This was very discouraging. At that point I wondered if it had been smart to come back. Until I wrote those mid-terms, I didn't know how I was doing. I thought I had fixed all of my past mistakes. I had a balanced course selection, reduced course load, contact with cooperative professors, and permission to write my exams in a private setting with extra time. I had good tutors and support people. It still wasn't enough.

What was going on? Could I improve? I had to change how I was studying. There was no other choice. I met with my professors to see if, and how, I could improve.

I really lucked out with my sociology professor. He was very accommodating and he knew a lot about learning disabilities. He had been a resource teacher in a high school before he became a professor. He suggested that we meet at least once a week during his office hours to discuss class lectures and any other questions that I had. I agreed to prepare chapter summaries of the readings for these meetings. I also agreed to attend the other section of his course, so that I would hear the lectures twice. We worked together on different methods of accommodation for that subject.

The big thing with sociology turned out to be that I had been trying to memorize everything and my memory for details is not that great. I found it very beneficial to try to understand the concepts and discuss the ideas with my professor. Doing summaries of everything we were covering as we went along was really useful. My marks showed the difference. By Christmas, my mark had gone from 53 per cent to 83 per cent.

In English, the professor just suggested that I focus on getting my novels read. He told me not to worry about getting the assignments handed in by the due dates. He knew that it was taking me extra time to get and to use the taped texts. I had taken an English class from him before and we both felt that I could do well in this course. I never missed a class. I thought about the material and I always participated in discussions. He reassured me that concentrating on doing a thorough job with the reading would allow the rest to follow. He was right. By the end of the year, I had earned an eighty-five.

In math, it was a bit different. The format for the calculus class had changed since I had first taken it. The program changes made the course more accommodating for people with different learning styles. At the end of each week there were quizzes. That timing helped me to summarize my notes for the week and my scores showed me my progress. The quizzes were also a big help in preparing for midterms and exams. I knew where I had to spend more time and I already had a lot of studying done. You could explain your answers using diagrams. There wasn't so much emphasis on getting the right answer. Showing your reasoning could give you some marks, even if you didn't get the right answer. We were also assigned a project. This was new. I love projects and I made full marks on mine, so that improved my average. All of this worked to my advantage.

The math professor advised me to read the textbook and do more examples. He said I really had to keep up with the class and stay on top of all of the material. Reading the text book and doing more problems helped my mark in several ways. I learned to pick a few questions on each topic and check them against the answers that were already available in the text. If I couldn't get them, I could ask for a step by step explanation. In previous years I just started at the beginning, and tried to do every question over and over until I got the right answer. It didn't take long to fall behind that way. I was now getting at least a little bit of practice with everything and not just dismissing my mistakes as careless little errors in order to move on.

It may seem strange that I wouldn't have read the textbook until the professor told me directly to do it, but throughout high school we never read the math text. You would just do exercises, blank to blank. What was the purpose of reading the textbook? Besides, reading was a problem for me. It wasn't until it was really stressed by the professor that I did it and with a reduced course load I had time to read. I was keeping up, so if I didn't understand the example that they gave in the textbook, I was able to ask questions. I would actually have something to ask in class. Other years I always went to review classes, but I would be there and not really know what to ask. I went to those classes because I thought maybe sitting in and listening to everyone else's questions might be of some help. At the very least it would show that I was trying. In the end it was confusing and made me feel even further behind.

I guess another big change was actually asking questions in class. That was very, very important to my success in calculus. Before I felt very inferior and stupid when I asked questions. The class was mainly younger, first year students. I thought that since I was older, I should be smarter. I guess the smartness would have come in being smart enough to ask questions. After that first midterm I started to ask questions. I know it helped. I got sixty-five on the Christmas calculus exam and I felt there was still room for improvement.

When the marks came in, I felt I had finally found what I needed to do to succeed. My overall average at Christmas exams was seventy-one per cent. I was relieved and ready to do more. I decided to see if I could take geometry, a required course for the education program. It was only offered every other year and I had taken the course before. My roommate was going to be in the class and I knew that he would be an excellent tutor for me. I wanted to try it even though at the time of my readmission I had been advised not to take more than one math course per term. Calculus was a prerequisite and I was just halfway through that course. My counsellor didn't approve, but I convinced the math department and the Dean's Office to give me permission under the condition that I would drop the course by the mid-point if it ended up being a problem.

Second term my marks got better in all of my classes, even though I had added another course. Geometry was as challenging as it had been the first time around, but this time I knew what the professor was talking about. I think that it did help my self-esteem to take that course. I knew that I could do it. I was able to get a respectable 60 per cent and say, "There, that's out of the way!"

At final exams I did very well. I ended up with a 76.4 per cent average. This pleased me very much. It was high enough for the Dean's List for achievement, instead of for probation. I felt well on my way to finishing my degree. Just seven more courses and I could graduate.

Although I didn't really want to be playing a time game again, I thought it would be nice if I could finish in May of the following year. Financially and for me as a person, it would be the best thing. This would allow me to apply to the education program for a September start. Summer courses could make this possible. If I took enough summer courses, I could also have a reduced course load in the fall and winter term. The course offerings weren't ideal and they kept changing. This made it impossible to get taped texts on time. The time frame was short and the work intense. I had never taken a course in this format before. My counsellor didn't approve of me taking three courses. She was very worried that I was taking on too much and starting to repeat the strategies that got me into difficulties in the past. In the end, I took two and a half courses over the summer term.

The time passed quickly. I learned to be very disciplined. I had to be, to keep up with the pace. In a way, I had a reduced load because I didn't do anything else. I had no job, no friends around, nothing but studying. As the weather got warmer I really wanted to be doing nothing, or at least not sitting in a classroom and studying. I had some rent and roommate problems. I learned that I really have to be focused for exams no matter how well I know the material. I get very nervous in exams, so I really need to take the time to go back over the material to reassure myself. Overall my marks were respectable, especially since the learning conditions were not ideal for me. It wasn't my best summer, but I completed two and a half more credits.

Year Six: Finishing My Degree

Just four and a half courses left to complete before I can graduate. It's exciting and scary all at the same time. It's more than last year, but I think I have chosen courses where I can balance my work load and be successful. It even gives me a course reduction for the second term.

I am looking forward to the year. This time I am not naive. I know that I have a lot of work to do. Hopefully, with the courses I have chosen, it won't be as difficult as in previous years. I know that I have to stay focused. I am getting a head start. I already have my English textbooks and all of my novels on tape. I am reading those before the term starts. I haven't ever done that before. I hope starting on the right foot is one more thing that will help to make me successful. I need another good year to continue on to the education program. I am still determined to achieve my original goal. I have dreamed about being a teacher for a very long time.

The Ingredients for Success

I think the critical ingredient for my success at university was realizing what a person with learning disabilities can achieve with goals and proper accommodation. I can see now that for much of my time at university I was working against my learning disability, not with it. Rather than thinking about how I could accommodate my learning pattern to reach my goals, I took the attitude that I couldn't do some things. I tried to avoid my learning disability. I didn't really look at how I learned. It was very short-term thinking. I look back now and it seems so simple. There were so many small things to change and to try that made a big difference, but back then I couldn't see them.

Having a learning disability in itself makes you feel different than everyone else. You feel that you have to try to make yourself seem so-called normal. You want to be like the other students that don't have a learning disability. You try to keep the pace of everyone else so that you don't appear odd. I didn't want to do anything that seemed odd. I didn't want to think of myself as needing something special like a reduced course load. I felt that would mean that I couldn't obtain all of my courses like everyone else. I was hurrying and trying so hard to be what I thought was normal that I wound up with two disastrous years and a year waiting to return to try again.

Now I believe that I am like everyone else. Everyone has problems and they have to adapt to deal with them. A learning disability is just like any other problem. Trying to deny that it's there is no solution. You have to seek out ways to work with it instead of against it. That took me a long time to sort out for myself. Sometimes I would overestimate my abilities. Sometimes I would underestimate them. Sometimes I was just lying to myself or being pig-headed. A perfect example would be any one of those math courses that I talked my way into without the prerequisites. I would walk into an exam with a twenty or a thirty average. I would tell myself, "Sure, you'll do well in the exam and pass this course." It just wasn't possible. Now I would recognize the problem earlier on and work toward fixing it. Now I would step back and ask: "Is this course for me? Should I be doing it now? What steps can I take to help me get through this course? How much time would they take? Is it possible for me to do this? What is the professor's view? What are the other options?" Now I would, but not then.

I never told people about my doubts. I always put up a very positive front. I think a person's outlook and attitude makes a big difference in the way people perceive you and treat you. I think there were many teachers who just gave me a pass because of the way I appeared to them. I think sometimes professors encouraged me and let me take courses even when I shouldn't have because of who I was. They thought I was a nice person. I had problems. They didn't want to make my life tougher, so they just let me do what I wanted to do.

After my second disastrous year, I did a new assessment of my learning style with my counsellor. This gave me confidence in my abilities. Discussing the test results helped me to see that I wasn't so-called 'stupid' in everything. I did have strengths. I had scores that were in the superior range. I am good at abstract reasoning and problem solving. I am good at picking up themes and meanings. I love mathematics, projects and presentations. I usually have a novel idea or way of presenting material that gets people's attention and I can pass along my enthusiasm. I love spending time on projects and presenting what I've done. The amount of work doesn't bother me. I always get good results. I think all of these things would make me a good teacher.

Although you may hope that there are areas of your ability that outweigh the areas where you are weak, there are many times when you are doubtful. It's easy to think, "I'm not good at this, so how could I possibly be good at any other subject or skill." After that assessment, I could talk about and think about my learning disability in a different way. I felt that I had a realistic picture of my strengths and weaknesses. Although that realistic picture did not make me entirely happy in the short term, I knew that it could help me succeed, and that it would make me happy in the long run.

Another big breakthrough was starting to try different types of accommodations, instead of just being afraid and avoiding things that I thought learning disabled students couldn't do. When I finally got the nerve to try an English course, it was my highest grade. Achieving good marks in courses using different types of accommodations made a big impression on me. I started working more with the professors to find the right learning style and accommodation for each of the courses. When all of the right ingredients were there, I saw my marks go from fifty-three to eighty-three. Now I feel that I could tell you about my learning disability and how to accommodate for it at university, in a way that just was not possible for a very long time. It's a long list, but it doesn't overwhelm me anymore.

To be successful at university, I accommodate for my learning style in a number of ways. I have a notetaker in lectures to make sure I don't miss a concept and to make sure that terms are spelled correctly. Before I had notetakers I would be struggling over getting the main words down. I would miss the definition or the point of the issue discussed. If terms aren't spelled correctly, it is very hard for me to learn the names and vocabulary of the course. I have to put extra time into rehearsing names and key terms in each course. Sometimes I use flashcards or other visual aids. Sometimes I just try to work around using the term or the name. I have special notetaking paper that allows my notetaker to take notes and have a copy for me as well. That way there is no inconvenience.

I also use taped texts. Having my books on tape allows me to listen and follow along with the print at the same time. That way I don't have to concentrate on trying to make out the words and trying to take in what the text is actually saying. I am able to concentrate on the information and the meaning. With practice I have learned to use the tapes much more efficiently. I can 'read' the four-track tapes at chipmunk-speed now.

For tests and exams, I need to work in a private setting. I get very anxious and I'm easily distracted. It helps to have the proctor read the exam questions to me, in case I have missed or misunderstood words. When I hear the questions, or when I hear my own answers read out, they often seem quite different than what I have understood from the print. I also like to read out loud to myself as I work on an answer. It helps me to get organized. I like to prepare my answers on the computer, so that I can use the spell check. It's easy to read when I'm done, and it's also very good for revising and organizing answers. For some exams I put my answers on a dictaphone and then they are typed for submission to the professor. With math I just do the best I can with the quiet setting and some extra time. There is usually not the same amount of print involved in a math exam. The option I choose usually depends on the type of course, the kind of the testing and the professor's preference.

I take a reduced course load. It gives me the extra time that I need to do the accommodations I require. Before having a reduced course load, I could work from the moment I got home from class to the time I went to bed at one or two o'clock in the morning and still not achieve what I needed to get done. Sometimes I wouldn't even get half of the work done that I needed for the next day. Just as in exams, it takes me extra time to use the aids I need.

It took me a long time to learn to use my time wisely. I had to learn how to use accommodation techniques effectively. I don't need the same thing for every course. I've learned how to work with tutors and professors to get the support and teaching that I need. I have learned to ask myself: Will I really use this accommodation? Do I have time to use it? Is there any other method I could use? I've learned when I actually need notetakers. Although tapes of lectures and taped texts hadn't worked very well for me at the start, I found better ways of using them. Then they definitely became worth the time. Using taped texts has allowed me to take courses that I otherwise would have had to avoid.

My sociology course is a good example. Instead of having a notetaker, I attended a second session of the class. I found that a better way to use my time. The second presentation of the material was better than reading notes and trying to incorporate them into my own version of the lecture. The extra three hours spent each week in the lectures was also more interesting than re-reading notes or listening to a tape of the lecture. There were different questions asked and additional discussion. My knowledge and understanding of what was going on in class was expanded.

I also started using a priority system. Instead of trying to schedule everything in, I decided what was most important to get accomplished and did that. By the end of the year the reading in sociology had increased to the point that I didn't have time to use the taped texts. Instead I just skimmed the print for the key words and spent my time on completing the summaries of key topics. I discussed my summaries with the professor or another student once each week. I listened to the priorities stressed by the professor. I kept in contact to make sure that I was on the right track. I was able to figure out myself how to cut corners and make the best use of my time. This is entirely different from starting at the beginning, trying to do everything and falling more behind all the time. That's what I used to do. With a priority system the results are much better and there's much less stress.

It was a long struggle for me to learn all of this. Even now I may not always be able to do things the way I know I should, but at least I know what I am capable of doing under learning conditions that suit my style. The other long struggle is to educate the professors, tutors and all of the people at a university, so that they really understand what a learning disability is. We all learn differently and they all need to learn to take the time to find out specifically what each person's learning style is. Hopefully they will have open minds and take in what the student is telling them. Then they can respond with some helpful suggestions. If there is more community education people will realize that a learning disability is a real and complicated thing. It is not a figment of someone's imagination.

It was extremely helpful to me to have discussions with the professors. I needed to be able to talk about how I learned and how I could learn more effectively. I needed professors to be really honest with me and say what they thought as a professor about the problems they could foresee with their course. I needed their advice on possible solutions. Although they may not think of themselves as the nice professor by telling students that they can't achieve something, sometimes it is exactly what the student needs to hear. Working with the professors helped me in two ways. It allowed me to reach down, assess my strategies and honestly decide, "Can I do the things I need to do to even have a chance at being successful?" Sometimes I just couldn't accept what the professor was saying and it made me work harder to prove that I could succeed. Either way, it was a help.

I don't think this understanding and communication about learning disabilities is an easy thing to accomplish, but I think it is a critical ingredient for success. Both the students with the learning disabilities and the people around them need to realize what persons with learning disabilities can achieve, and what is needed to achieve success. No one will tell you that it is easy for someone with a learning disability to succeed at university, but it is important for everyone to know that it is possible.

As I said at the start, my time at university has definitely had its ups and downs, but I never gave up. It may take me longer to get there, but when I'm there no one can take my university degree away from me. I am on my way to a teacher training program. I am many steps

158   *Learning Disabilities and Success*

closer to accomplishing my dream. Remember, having a learning disability doesn't mean you can't accomplish your dream.

THE VIEW FROM OUTSIDE

I first met Alice when she came to our transition workshop for high school students with learning disabilities. Her positive nature and her enthusiasm for university studies stood out immediately. She seemed comfortable with people and very capable. In addition to participating in our workshops, she arranged a residence tour on her own and selected her accommodation for the fall. I was impressed by her independence and her initiative. She was very clear about her educational goals. She wanted to be a teacher, with math and business as her specialty. She seemed well organized to begin her studies at university. She certainly didn't plan to let the idea of being a student with a learning disability stop her.

Alice's learning disability had been diagnosed when she was in grade two. Since that time, she had participated in special needs programming. She had strong support from her family and a resource teacher in her high school. She was very active in her church and in her community. She tutored children in mathematics and had developed a small sales business following the junior achievement model. Even though school had been difficult for her, she had found ways of making a positive contribution. Alice was admired for her resourcefulness, her hard work and her generosity. Her diagnostic testing indicated that she had above average ability in areas valued in university studies, but that she was severely learning disabled. She needed to use the full range of services available to assist her in learning and demonstrating her mastery of course content. It would not be easy, but all of the ingredients seemed to be there for success.

As you know from reading her story, it did not turn out to be easy at all. Her time at university ends up providing us with a picture of both success and failure, as Alice learns how to work "with her learning disability, not against it." The difference in the way she describes her experiences in her first few years at university, compared with the range and control of strategies she eventually learns to use, is dramatic. Alice was determined to prove that her learning disability couldn't stop her from being a normal worthwhile person. That focus led her to university and to a denial of the deficits that she carried along with her strengths. Once she gained confidence in an integrated view of her learning strengths and weaknesses, she was able to redirect her energies and reach the goals she treasured.

Alice's struggles reveal how difficult it is to deal with a mixed pattern of abilities and the confusing feedback that results. Formal grades and evaluations have presented Alice with a varied and changing picture of her ability and her potential. Advice and support from other people is similarly mixed. It is hardly surprising that Alice struggled with overestimating and underestimating her abilities. To add to this confusion, Alice did not wish to be seen as disabled. Clearly she is very able in many areas. She is a creative thinker and can find her way through complex problem situations. She is such a persuasive negotiator that she has talked herself into and out of many impossible situations.

In many ways the world simply did not make sense to Alice. She did not value or trust any of the grades she had received in her earlier schooling. For all of her school life she had been in programs for children who couldn't succeed, yet here she was at university. She liked the outcome, but she had no fundamental knowledge of the intellectual strengths that had made this possible and a worthwhile choice. She had been rewarded, both inside and outside of school, for her personal strengths. To Alice that seemed real. Now that she was at university people were taking her seriously as a student, perhaps for the first time, and she was overwhelmed by the deficits that stood in her way. All she had to defend herself were her impressive personal qualities, and a faith and desire that would not let her quit.

Instead of exposing her worries and fears about her ability to succeed, she used a positive attitude to convince herself and others that success was imminent. This strategy was only reassuring in the short run. Her own doubts and worst fears about her ability, combined with her determined optimism, pushed her into denying the reality of her situation. Tastes of success seemed to encourage Alice to disregard her weaknesses altogether and deny herself the use of strategies that allowed her to express her abilities. She attributed many of her successes to people being nice or to luck, while attributing her failure to factors beyond her control. Her upbeat comments tried to suggest that she had things under control with a new strategy that couldn't fail. She rushed over the negative feedback that came her way, and began to feel that people were rewarding her for her hard work and personal qualities rather than her ability, just as they had in high school. For much of her time at university Alice relied on good will, luck and perseverance as a survival technique, rather than developing effective strategies to deal with her learning situation.

I have to admit that I was a long time catching on to this pattern. I met regularly with Alice and she dazzled me with the details of her week and her plans. I was reassured by her cheerful approach, her many activities and her resistance to adversity. I liked and admired her. It never occurred to me that she doubted her own abilities and had not come to terms with her disability. When I came back from my leave year, I was surprised to find that Alice was in academic difficulties. I would have predicted just the opposite. She seemed to have a good base to build on from her first year, but instead she was on probation. She was suffering from a series of losses in her personal life and now she was also trying to cope with academic failure as well. Alice's response to her lack of success was to take on more courses and activities to make up for her failures, rather than slowing down and regrouping. She was going to catch up and solve the problem with hard work. The negative spiral just deepened. The more desperate her situation, the more she refused to adjust. It was as if all she had left was her determination and she was clinging to it.

Even Alice's enthusiasm and desire to be a teacher was working against her. She was already teaching mathematics to young children who were struggling with the subject in school. Ever since high school, she had taught Sunday school and made her spending money tutoring. In practice she was a teacher. This gave her confidence, but it also made her impatient for affirmation and accreditation. Taking a lighter course load and a slower route was an impossible choice for Alice, even though experience was showing her that it might be the most efficient approach in the long run.

At one of these dark moments, while she was waiting to appeal her dismissal, I suggested we should revisit her assessment and get a picture of her abilities from another source. We did some new testing together and then we discussed her learning profile. Alice was relieved. Her high scores gave her confidence. The results made sense to her and they gave her a new way to approach learning. Now she knew that she had more than social skills and structural supports available to manage her learning situation. It took intense pressure to make her stop and take another look at what she could and could not do. I think this time-out was the beginning of progress. Her time away from university allowed her to rebuild her confidence and develop some of the basic skills she needed. Alice's new vision of herself and her abilities gave her the tools to develop the working partnerships she needed with her professors. Her poor marks on the first set of midterms made her take the risk. Her new awareness and understanding of her learning disability gave her the ability to hear and use feedback in a way that opened the possibility of success.

It took time for all of the changes Alice needed to make to be sorted out, but the pieces started fitting together. She came to terms with both her strengths and weaknesses as a learner. As her counsellor, I had sometimes found her struggles difficult to watch. Alice and I often disagreed, but we always maintained a strong connection. It was easy to respect her willingness to take on a challenge and her desire to do well, but it was very frustrating to see those positive qualities work against her. Alice has now mastered a complex set of learning skills and has the confidence and flexibility to use them effectively. Along the way she has taught me and many other people at the university, a great deal about learning and teaching.

Alice had the courage to follow her dream and work through the failures that involved. At times it seemed an almost impossible task. Along the way she has given many hours of her time to help us develop a better system for students with disabilities and she has been a kind and generous friend to many. In the time that has passed since our interviews, Alice has had her moments on the Dean's List and earned both her Bachelor of Arts degree and a Bachelor's degree in education. She is now an accredited teacher. No one doubts her spirit, strength and determination and the lessons she can teach about accomplishing your dream.

Postscript: From Alice to Sophie Rose

Over the years, I lost touch with Alice. I can tell you that after she graduated with her Bachelor of Education degree, she took a position teaching in an isolated northern community. The happy beginnings of a dream come true did not have the outcome we all hoped for. Alice was not able to manage a full-time classroom position. She experienced health problems and she returned to our university town. Alice made the best of her situation and set up a service offering tutoring and math camps for kids. This option had worked well for her in the past. I know she wanted more but with reduced stress her health improved. Alice remained active in her church. At a summer retreat, she met her future partner. They married and moved some distance away to work together in their faith community. I cannot tell you more of her life after university. From her past history, I can't imagine that Alice would give up on her dream even if it meant having to find a non-traditional way to be a teacher. I like to think she is out there, passing on her love of mathematics, helping her family and her community and finding satisfaction in doing it.

In Alice's place I have invited Sophie Rose, another veteran of our Speakers' Bureau, to contribute her story. Both Sophie and Alice had a long-held dream of being a teacher and a strong desire to make things better for children in schools. They were the kind of people who are labelled 'born teachers'. Even before graduating from university, each had earned respect and employment in teaching roles in their own communities. In Alice's case she was tutoring math and running summer camps along with managing a junior achievement business. Sophie coached sports and taught swimming and figure skating. In the summers she managed the local recreation center.

For both of these young women, having a career in teaching and having a family were sustaining goals. Their dreams and determination led them to pursue teaching qualifications at university. Though each had struggled at university, they both succeeded in earning a teaching degree. As it turned out they also shared many frustrating and discouraging experiences in their attempts to be employed in a local school. They were challenged to find other pathways to meaningful careers. While recognizing the differences in the two stories, I think their commonalities make Sophie's experiences of life after university a helpful companion to Alice's story.

9
Sophie Rose
World of Work

I met with Sophie at her home in the rural community where she grew up. She and her husband have built a spacious home on waterfront property with breathtaking views. I could certainly see how the beauty of the setting could capture you. Sophie's parents live on the neighbouring lot. Having family nearby is an important bonus in this sparsely populated countryside. Inside, Sophie has created a warm, comfortable and well-ordered environment that both adults and children can enjoy. As she pointed out, this was all part of her plan. Her son is off at the parent-run co-op daycare where Sophie volunteers. She took time away from her morning duties so we could talk undisturbed. As always, Sophie is lively and enthusiastic in conversation. We laughed a lot, especially about her frustrations past and present. Humour is definitely a big part of the way Sophie maintains her balance, especially in the face of difficult times. I was reminded of the way she had both charmed and inspired audiences as part of our Speakers' Bureau. Here is her story.

I Have a Plan

I am thirty-eight years old and I graduated from university with a Bachelor's Degree in Human Kinetics and a Bachelor's Degree in Education. It was hard, but I did it. A lot of things have happened since I graduated. I've married and with my partner we've moved back to our home community, built a house on the water near my parents, and had children. This was all part of the plan my husband and I have had since we were young.

My partner and I have been together for a very long time. We grew up together. When we were young, we were going through a lot of the same situations in school but my husband would never say he had a learning problem. After high school he went to community college and learned a skilled trade. Now he has a good job and he is good at it. He is never without work. Because of my husband's job, we were able to build the house and live here where we want to be. I'm lucky. I don't know a lot of people my age who can say that.

Another part of the plan was that I would be a teacher here at the local school. Even though I had a lot of negative experiences in school, I always expected to go to university and become a teacher. I grew up teaching swimming and figure skating. I coached sports teams and managed the recreation program for the summer. I liked teaching. I knew I was good at it because I got great feedback and people kept hiring me back. I don't think I really had the Oprah-ness to have an Ah-ha moment and know "I can achieve that." Maybe now I might. Back then it seemed simple. I wanted to be a teacher so I went to university. My parents never pressured me into going. I just thought that's what I needed to do to have the career I wanted.

I guess the thing is that in some ways, I wanted to educate the teachers as much as the kids. I know what it's like to be sitting in a desk not understanding and getting frustrated. I wasn't a kid to lash out or do anything like that. I never really said anything to complain. I never, ever even said "I don't understand" when the teacher asked, "Does anyone not understand?" Who the hell is going to put their hand up then? I thought I would be a teacher who would help those kids like me.

I think I would be an excellent physical education teacher or ideally I'd love to be teaching in a learning centre. I don't really see myself in a big elementary classroom with thirty kids. I see myself sitting around a table with a smaller group and helping them figure out how to find success at school. I wanted to be in a place to help the kids who are struggling. The only problem is that I couldn't seem to convince the people who do the hiring to make that possible. The school teaching part of the plan hasn't worked out so well.

Believe me, for about four years after getting my university degrees I tried everything I could think of to get that teaching job back home. I know there are other places that value physical education and alternative approaches, but that was just not happening in my area. It was a very frustrating and stressful period. I started to doubt myself. I'm glad I had other things going for me at the same time. It took me a while to accept that there are many ways to teach without having to be in a box in a school. I had worked for so long toward that goal and it meant so much to me, that it was very hard to step back and look at other opportunities.

Eventually, it became obvious to me that if I was going to stay in my home community and have a career, I would have to explore some other options. After those years of frustration, I realized that at the end of the day I am a person who likes to help others and there are many ways to do that. I know now that it's not necessary to be standing in a classroom behind a desk to teach life skills or to be helpful to people. I've made some adjustments to the plan and it's working out pretty well.

Getting My Teaching Qualifications

The first part of the plan was getting to university. In my community some people just go to school and don't think too much about it. They get their grade twelve or maybe they don't get their grade twelve. It doesn't matter. But the gang that I ran with wanted to go to university. That's what you did and what I saw my brother do. Both my mother and father have been to university at some point too. There was a time when me, my father and my brother were all in university at the same time. My parents must have eaten Kraft Dinner for a long time to get us all there. I didn't give community college a thought. Their program in recreation management might have been a good option for me but the only places I applied after high school were universities. Now my brother and I say, "What were we thinking?" Everyone we know who went to community college has a job, and is making lots of money, and we're both poorly employed teachers .... silly, silly people.

Until I went to university, I really didn't know that I had what people called a "learning disability". I had an appointment at the university before I started classes but I didn't realize it was with the Program for Students with Disabilities. Those words came out of someone's mouth and I thought "Hey, they are talking about me." Maybe nowadays I would have known but I really didn't then. I just thought that I was not great at reading and writing. I didn't know that meant a learning disability. It turns out that of the grandkids in my family, eight of us have learning disabilities. I totally think my father has a learning disability. We write and read exactly alike. There were so many people in my life that have trouble with reading and writing and spelling that it wasn't any big deal. We just got on with things.

Now I realize it's not like that for everyone. Once, when I was substitute teaching at a high school, a student came to me and said "I can't do that. I have dyslexia." I said "So what? Yes, you can do it. You've just got to figure out *how* you can do it." I was surprised at the student's comment and the student wasn't ready for my answer. She was ready to give up and all that she wanted was my consent.

Amazing! I'm glad my parents always expected me to get out there and participate. They helped me figure out how I could. They had confidence in me and made me feel that I could succeed even if it meant lots of hard work.

Accommodating My Learning Style

I don't know if it made a difference to me that no one put a label on the way I learned. I just knew that my mom had a lot of meetings at the school and I knew that it took me a long time to do things. I wasn't one of those people who could just sit in the room and hear something and then automatically remember it for the next exam. I had friends around me that weren't like that either but I always copied notes from those friends that were quick and had good marks. I even moved in with some of them in the first year of university. I don't know how that happened. I was probably coaxed in the right direction.

I've always tried to create some sort of support circle. At high school it would be a couple of the smart people in my class. I would try to be friends with them. I didn't do it on purpose. It just happened that way. We were friends from sharing notes. I would go to them and copy their notes so I would have notes to study for the tests. Some people might have thought that I was being lazy but I did take my own notes too. With the learning disability that I have, I would get hung up on a certain word. I would be stuck on that word like a bouncy ball until I could figure out how to spell it. Meanwhile the teacher kept going so then I had missed the whole paragraph. It didn't make any sense to leave that word unfinished because, when I looked back at the end of the day, I would never remember what it should be. I would have to try to figure it out. If you had my notes and my friends' notes you could see where I got some of the information but not all of it.

I don't know if the two people I got information from understood the way I learned or not. My parents were friends with their parents. With one of them, we were involved in everything together ever since we were little. This would be everything inside and outside of school. We both did sports and lots of extra school activities. In this community, if you go to daycare with someone, then you go to primary and then you're with that person until grade twelve. Most of the time there was just one class of every grade so we were always together. That was a good thing and it could be a bad thing. You had the outspoken kid who liked to argue or some kids with behavioral issues and you were stuck with them all the time. I was good at the social side of school. I was often a leader or organizer in school events. I had lots of friends and lots of fun. I don't think people paid much attention to how I was doing in academics except for my parents.

At high school, if you needed extra help you could get it during the lunch break. We always had an hour off at lunch time. They had activities then too. For someone like me, who was active in everything and needed to be, there was no way I would ever go for extra help at lunch. I always had to do something for volleyball or yearbook or students' council or whatever. We used to have that conversation with the teachers and ask them to stay after school. Most of them had to travel over an hour to get to us and there was no way they felt they could add extra time to their day at the school. Some of the teachers that lived in the area were willing to help. They had a better understanding of what students here were up against. At one point someone's father was tutoring a bunch of us in math at the kitchen table in the evenings. The community came to our rescue and found a way for us to get what we needed. The extra help with that father was the only reason I passed math class.

I didn't know why at the time but my mom would push me into the more academic classes in high school. Obviously my parents had a bigger plan for my education that I didn't figure out until later. My mom insisted that I take my classes in French, because she knew that those kids had education as a higher priority than the kids who picked shop or tourism. She wanted me in French, not because it was especially important to her for me to learn the language, but because of the students that were in that class.

Unfortunately, French was a terrible class for me. I didn't understand English let alone how to deal with another language. My mom didn't understand when I wanted to quit that class. She was pretty upset but so was I. When I was older I understood why she wanted me there, but at the time I couldn't understand why she was torturing me like that. And she didn't stop with just French class. She put me in core French so that I had all of my subjects in French. She felt that, given the choices available, it was the best option for me. It's not that my parents were hard-core scary people. In most ways their high expectations were good for me. They wanted me to get a good education that would take me beyond high school.

In my mind, this decision about French led to behavioural issues for me in class. Not that I was crazy out there but obviously I didn't have an attention span to cope in class. I had no idea what they were talking about. I assume I was passing French but I don't know how. Luckily the teacher was transferred and they couldn't offer core

French anymore. That was how in grade eleven I finally got my way and returned to English. Socially school was always good for me. I got lots of praise for the extra-curricular stuff I did. That made up for the other parts. One way or another I managed to qualify for university.

My University Years

Even though I had my trials at high school, university was a lot more work and a lot less fun. What was frustrating was how hard I worked, especially in my first year. I identified myself as learning disabled to my professors. I knew I had to but I did it more in a passive way. I was still trying to figure out what I needed. For me year one seemed to be all about paper work. To get the accommodations and equipment I needed there was always paperwork involved. I had to sort out how to get class notes down. Then there was trying to get the papers done for my courses. I worked like I did in high school and it wasn't enough. At the end of the year I was half a point away from the average I needed to come back.

Never did I ever think that I was going to fail out, even though I was getting mid-terms and assignments back and I wasn't passing. I thought, if I was sitting in that study hall and I wasn't partying, I was doing what I was supposed to do. I was living off campus and had a quiet place to work. I went to every class. I was working hard. I was like the little engine going up the hill. I just thought the ducks were in a row and it was going to turn out right. In first year, I only passed one assignment and that was with a fifty-three. There was no way I could ever keep up with the reading and the paperwork. No wonder I failed out! But I didn't clue in until the final marks arrived.

How could it have gone so wrong? I came to university with the students who were my support system in high school. They were in my house but I didn't rely on them like I did in high school. For one thing, they were in different courses. I know now it was weird to think this way but I didn't want to open my mouth and say anything to anyone. It's not how I usually am. I tried talking with one professor and he said to me, "I think this learning disability is all in your head. I think this is something you can get over." It was like I had a disease or a sickness and I could just take some Advil and I'd be okay and would be able to pass his class. Believe it or not this was my psychology professor. Wow! I guess I'm hoping that some new teachers and some new professors are filtering some of these people out. I'd like to think that the times have changed for the better as far as understanding about learning disabilities is concerned.

I was hauled into the Dean's office after the first set of mid-terms. I had failed them all. They wanted me to explain why this was happening. I knew people who had failed out. It was because they were drinking and they weren't going to class and other things. I remember sitting in the waiting room where they gave me a survey to fill out. How many hours do you party a week? I put zero and I'm sure they thought it was hilarious. I just said listen, this is what's going on. I described what I was doing. They probably didn't believe me. I didn't! I think I must have been the only frosh that didn't participate in all of that craziness. I knew I couldn't go to parties and do those crazy things and still function the next day. I knew I had to be sitting in my bedroom and reading. How could it not be working?

I think those final marks opened my eyes. Technically I had failed out. I was determined that I wasn't going back home. It was never an option in my head. It was expected that after high school, I would do something more. My parents thought so and I did too. Those final marks made me realize that if I wanted to stay, I actually had to get it together and deal with my learning disability. I appealed to the committee on studies and they agreed to let me come back and try.

Finding My Way

After this hoopla happened with my marks, I knew I had better open my mouth and speak up. I also had to figure out what I needed. I know I can organize things, but if you don't have the lecture notes to organize, then how can you memorize them? That's when I started to use the Centre for Students with Disabilities more often. By then I had my technology too and I learned how to use it. The way I managed at university really changed. I knew it had to.

Getting good notes was always important for me. I started tape recording some of my lectures. Some of them, like human kinetics, made sense even without taping. Some professors were good about putting things online and giving out handouts. One professor must have killed about a thousand trees. All of her lectures were in a package. You still had to go to class because you would miss things, but you had a base to follow along and add comments. I also had the special carbon paper to give to a note taker for producing my notes. In history, my cousin took some of the same classes as me. I would get a copy of her notes. She wrote like crazy so I got very complete notes from her.

For exams I was in a private room with a reader and for some I didn't need one. I remember a lot of the multiple-choice tests where they would try to stump you. I had a reader for those and some of the biology courses. Sometimes the reader was allowed to spell the word for me. When I was taking anatomy and physiology I could say the words but I could never spell them. I had a great tutor for that course and a reader who understood the terms. When you have a reader who doesn't know the terminology, it really is confusing to do the exam with them. My best reader would say the word the right way, then that would trigger my memory and I could remember the concept.

I also took a reduced course load to have more time to do everything I needed. I called it going on the five-year plan. The only thing about taking more than the usual four years was this mind-set from where I grew up. There you start and you finish with the same people. Everyone from home that I started with in university graduated the year before I did. At Christmas, I had enough credits to qualify for my grad-ring with the gang from home. I got to be part of the celebrations but I knew I had to come back for another year. I didn't like the way that made me feel. The year that I was supposed to graduate was kind of tough for me.

All along, my friends never knew I had failed out first year. I never told anybody. I just had a reduced course load. I was going along doing my thing. The gang probably still think I graduated with them because who knows or remembers all the details of other people's lives? It probably only bothered me. It made sense to take a reduced course load. I should probably have done that in my first year too but there's no way you could have convinced me of that at the time.

After my first year, university was better for me academically than high school. Even though I wasn't having fun and being social, I learned more and got the marks I needed. I'm very cautious and unsure at the start of anything new. The wall comes up and I usually say, "Oh no, I can't do that." Then some of the people on my support team will say, "Well, you've done things like that before, so you can again." Then I keep trying. After my first year I learned a bunch of things I could do to manage my situation. Since I already liked to have a plan, I started planning better for my course strategies and it worked out pretty well.

I wouldn't say I managed all of that on my own. The people at the student center helped find tutors and readers for some of my classes. The exam rooms and proctors were all handled for me. They helped me fill in forms and qualify for my technology. I saw new options and ways to get things done. It was totally different than my first year and so were my marks. Technology and a circle of support from home and university made it all work out. Every year there were bumps but I got better at handling the problems and the stress. I was learning things. I graduated with a Bachelor's degree in Human Kinetics. That was another step in the plan accomplished.

Becoming a Teacher

The next part was getting into the Education program so that I could go back home and teach. Applying to the program was especially hard. There was lots of competition. I really wanted to get in but I wasn't at all sure they would take a person with a learning disability like me. I knew that I had plenty of experience. I had done lots of teaching in swimming and skating and summer recreation programs. I did volunteer placements in some elementary classes and worked with day care kids. I participated in speakers panels about disabilities. I believed I was a good candidate for the education program. What I had trouble with was finding the right way to express on those forms why I was a good candidate. It felt like I had to write about a hundred different essays trying to figure out how to identify myself and my learning disability. That was one of those times when I didn't want people to think that I was trying to put up an excuse. I wanted them to know that this is what you're getting if you select me. The way I looked at it, I was putting all of my cards on the table.

In those application essays you always had to say why you wanted to become a teacher. To sell myself, I talked about different things that had happened to me throughout my education. I realized once I got into the program that most student teachers had a positive experience in school and that's why they wanted to become teachers. Negative is a scary word but a lot of the experiences I had were negative. I wanted to make things better for kids who were struggling like I did. I felt that I should go back and try to break the cycle for losing and failing kids. That was really important to me. It still is.

It turned out that my application worked. I did manage to sell myself and get into the education program I wanted. Once I got into the B. Ed. program I finally felt "This is what I can do. This is what I want to do." It was lots of work but it was the kind of work I could do. Finally I didn't need to write a huge paper on Beowulf. Instead, I got to set up units on Science and Physical Education. Perfect! My supervisors were supportive. They found me good practice teaching placements that fit with my interests in special education and physical education. I got good feedback from my placements in the classrooms and I graduated with a Bachelor of Education Degree. I was officially a teacher. The plan was working just fine and I was pretty excited about the next steps. I thought the hardest part was over.

Getting the Job

The next part of the plan was to get a job back where my partner and I grew up. We moved back home, got married and started building our house. We were getting ready to start a family. There were no vacancies in the local schools but I put my name on the list for substitute teaching. I did that until I went off on maternity leave. To show my ability and my commitment, I put in time volunteering where ever I could. I've chaperoned dances. I coached the volleyball team. I've done the family fun nights. As it turned out, I think I could have used all of those hours better with my little person and with my husband. Instead, I tried to prove how much I wanted a career in teaching.

Substitute teaching was really stressful. Being in the classroom with the students was the best part. I would go to school early for eight o'clock and hang out with the kids until class started. I would eat my lunch with the kids. Why I wanted to be a teacher was to help the kids but it's hard to stay out of the games that are going on behind the scenes. A lot of the times I would go to work and stay away from the other teachers. There's all that scheming to get another job. I don't know what it's called but it's like office politics. I wanted to try to stay out of that because you lose the connection with why you wanted to be there in the first place. You can totally see why, after years of that stuff, some teachers have no idea of why they are still there. Some of them get really cranky and I think it's because they are sucked into all that negativity.

By the end of my time on the substitute list, the principal would call me to his office and I never knew what it would be for. Sometimes the principal would call me in just because he wanted me to work a couple of days. Sometimes he'd call me in and take a big strip off me. I never knew what to expect. I just didn't feel like I was valued or that I was on my way to becoming a successful teacher. The offers to fill in kept coming, but when our little person came along I took my name off the substitute list.

Teaching positions would be posted. I would apply but I couldn't seem to get a full-time job in the local school. It was frustrating. I knew it was a tough time to be looking, but there were times when you just wanted to shake somebody a little bit. Then my mother would remind me that I spent seven years in university. I have a lot of education and a lot to offer. There are many teachers out there who are not teaching in the school system. They are doing other great things. Maybe I would have to find another way to have a career too. I didn't agree. I had a plan and I wanted to make it happen. I had worked very hard for those seven years to get my qualifications and I wasn't going to abandon my goal. I kept trying.

The whole world of trying to get a job as a teacher is actually a pretty frustrating topic for me. For the longest time I kept applying for full time jobs. I'm scared to even talk about those job interviews. I know I can charm an audience as a speaker but that's when I'm talking about what I want to talk about and I'm leading the conversation. When the hiring committee is leading the conversation with their four standardized questions, I find it hard to figure out how to sell myself. In the Education program they filled us with enthusiasm. Through those two years, we worked on those beautiful portfolios so we would be able to go in and highlight all our assets. But at the school board where I wanted to work, I get an essay and four set questions in the interview. This was not the best way for me to sell myself.

I have always identified my learning disability in my application. There is an actual box on the applications where you can identify it but there are no satisfactory accommodations. I have been given a computer to type up the essay portion of the interview but for someone like me, some extra time would be nice too. A forty-five minute time limit is not ideal. Luckily I had the scan and read pen. It was essential then because I couldn't afford to be stuck on a bouncy-ball word.

Then there was the interview. That process is crazy. I feel that the interview process is for a certain type and I'm not that type. You go in. You have just had forty-five minutes to write an amazing essay to try and sell yourself. Then you go for the interview where you're asked four set questions, this time in front of a panel and you have to try to sell yourself all over again. I can't do well under those conditions. But this is how they did it where I wanted to work.

After going for interview, after interview, after interview, I started to wonder is it the interview process or am I just an awful candidate? When I'm sitting there, I'm obviously not giving the right answers. One question where I always do well is talking about technology. I do know a lot about assistive technology and not that many people in our area do. Because of my background in kinetics and sports you would think I would be a good candidate for a position in physical education.

But those positions are really rare in our area, since physical education isn't a funding priority. One position that always keeps coming up here at the school is a learning centre position. I should be a natural for that but it's not happening. I couldn't seem to crack it. It was just hard. It would be great if you got feedback after the interview. That way you could figure out how to improve.

It feels like before you even sit in front of the hiring panel sixty percent of your interview is already done. It's based on your references, your application and the essay. That should be good for me. I have my fans and I've rehearsed my essay. I made sure the people that I listed for references were going to be positive, so that's not it. Sometimes the only person that I know on the panel is the principal, and then other times I know everybody. There was obviously something that was not working for me.

It got to the point that when I would go for a teaching interview I felt "I am not qualified. I'm not what they're looking for." I had a huge bag full of materials that I had collected to read and study to prepare for interviews. I might find out two days before an interview and then I would study to the point where I couldn't even eat the day of the interview. Then I would stress over the possibility that something would happen on the way to the interview and I wouldn't get there on time. I would leave about three hours before I needed to be there. Then I would sit in the parking lot reading my stuff over. It was just draining before the whole interview process even began. Then at the end of the day when I got back home, I would get the call saying "You are not the successful candidate."

That's when I would start to think "It's me. I'm not a good teacher. I just can't fit the mould." I forget that I don't want to fit that mould. It's hard to say "Well maybe it's them and not me." The first thing I do is think I'm the problem. Then I think "Do I really want to be there if it's that frustrating? What did I just bite off? I don't want it to be just a fight where I want to win the battle and then when I do win, it's not right and I don't want to be there anyway." It's was a vicious circle but I still applied for all the positions that came up. I wanted to get my name out there and show that I was still interested. I didn't want people to think I was just sitting here and happy doing nothing.

I tried tutoring. There was a kid who was suspended from school for a year and I was hired to tutor him. It wasn't a positive experience because it was high school level courses and it was material that I wasn't familiar with. The areas that are in demand for tutoring are math and physics and those are not areas where I am strong. For me to tutor privately, I would have to have all of that material and study it for a long time before I could teach it to somebody else. If it's not familiar material it just doesn't work. There would be a lot of hours of work and many of them would be at prime time for my own children. There is just no money in tutoring privately, especially in comparison to the school system.

I always put on my applications that I would be willing to take more specialized education. I know I could do more education even though I have children now. My mom studied special education when we were little even though she had to travel to do it. I applied for a master's program. I told the administrator at the Board, "I'm willing, I'm ready." She agreed. She thought I was a great candidate. I got accepted as a candidate by the local level but was declined by the university that offered the courses because I didn't have two years teaching experience. Hello! I can't get the teaching because I don't have the master's degree. I think that's what happens. People just get stuck on these silly details especially when there aren't many jobs. I felt like I was in one of those Looney Tunes cartoons where you're just spinning and you're the road runner, but you can't take off!

When I had the chance, I went to the professional development sessions in my area. I was sitting in on a presentation on inclusion for students with disabilities and a former teacher of mine was also there. He said to me "So you guys buy into this inclusion thing." He spoke as if inclusion was something that someone was trying to sell him, like a set of encyclopedia or something else he wouldn't want or need. I felt like shouting. Some people just think you're making a disability up and time has shown me that he isn't alone. I wanted a chance to break the cycle of negativity that kids who learn differently experience.

I would get pretty down after interviewing and getting the call to say I was unsuccessful. Once I was told that I had a great interview but the candidate that got the job over me had a position with the school board already, so she had to be selected. In that situation, I really didn't know what to think. I've had principals who know me from substitute teaching and they come to me and say, "I want you to apply for this position." But I still didn't get a job offer. I applied for a position where the principal and the vice principal and the person that was going off on leave handed me the teaching material to use when I started the job. I didn't get the position. People who know me would come to me and ask why I'm not teaching. It was just really hard on the head and it was frustrating! I don't know what else I could have done to show my ability and my commitment.

Sometimes I thought that it was my learning disability that kept me from getting a teaching position. Should I kick up a fuss about not being hired? Some days I would think about sticking up and saying something, but I was afraid making a complaint wouldn't be pretty. It probably wouldn't really help either. I knew a girl who couldn't get into the B.Ed. program so she kicked up a fuss and put this ridiculous article in the local paper. The next year, she got into the B.Ed. program. Making a fuss can work but I don't want to be known as the person that kicked up a fuss and then got a job. As far as the school board here is concerned, I don't know if my efforts would ever amount to anything anyway. We are losing population and this year there are thirty teaching jobs being cut back. It's crazy.

Revising the Plan

That was five years ago. I wanted to be home in my community no matter what. That wasn't going to change. Some days I didn't know what to do. Any jobs are scarce here. Everyone is in the same boat. A lot of us in my generation racked up a huge debt getting a university education. Now we are at home with our little ones and not in a career earning a big salary. I always say that women tend to work for the causes that make the most difference. They sit on boards for daycare or programs and activities for children but they're never paid for it. They are out there trying to fund-raise in their own way. Sometimes it's from bake sales or writing funding applications to get resources for the community. It's not only here though. But it is not the future I saw for myself after university.

Instead of being hung up on all of that, I decided to focus on the other things that I have in my life. I thought if I couldn't teach in a school maybe I could try teaching outside of school. I didn't want to try private tutoring again. I realized it would be best for me to run with things related to my strengths in sports and human kinetics. Some days I'm sorry I didn't take the fitness and personal trainer course at university but I was scared of the professor. When I was young I did figure skating and some coaching so it seemed a good thing to build on. I decided to work on qualifying to be a professional coach. I spent two years of training nights and weekends. I am now certified as a professional figure skating coach. Instead of travelling the roads to work at other arenas, I decided to try to build up a club here. Now I'm on the ice coaching eight hours a week for about 24 weeks of the year.

The numbers of students keep growing. We now have a club in our community and we've branched out to include teaching basic skating skills and holding family recreation events as well. We are a few years along and it's going well. Everybody around here looks forward to our Christmas Gala Show.

There's usually some contract work in the community for me to do. It seems every year they bring me back in May to organize and raise a crowd for our local folk festival. I'm there working until the festival is over at the end of the summer. It fits in after skating is over. I've worked for the festival since I was a student. I've moved on up the ladder from ticket sales. Right now I'm doing Artist Relations Management. Basically I facilitate bringing these artists in from all over the world. I make sure they have a place to stay and that they know what's going on and when. We sort out how they're going to get paid. I deal with a lot of details and complications. The festival is a big deal here. It's an annual event and it has a great reputation. The whole community gets a lot of benefit from it.

I also work with Early Childhood Intervention when they get some government funding to bring parent training or other programs to our community. Rural out-reach programs are an important resource for us and I have been interested in early intervention since I was a student. My mother has been a field worker with the provincial program for many years. I publicize, set up and facilitate the training session at the various locations. I do the tea and coffee too and cookies if we've got them.

Now I enjoy doing the contract stuff and the coaching a lot more than the thought of teaching in a school. I like to organize and I can do it well. It's easy for me. People see that and give you a pat on the back. It's nice to feel that appreciation. You know the old saying, "if you want something done, ask a busy person." So in my community I get asked a lot. There's no lack of opportunity for me to do things. But everything that's going on doesn't always reflect on the bank account. I am always busy but as far as earning money, not so much.

I started using the internet to widen my search for jobs. I used to dream that I might be able to work remotely. I thought that in a perfect world people wouldn't have to work away for days or weeks at a time like my husband does. Everyone could save themselves time away or an exhausting commute by working from home.

Well, I found that dream job. I've started an online business. It's based on a product line that I found on the internet for a skin condition I had developed (probably from changing too many diapers and doing too much housework). I have a deal with an international company. We sell product lines as part of a holistic wellness approach. It fits right in with things I learned at university and with my own experience. My business starts with a skin care focus but it is really about good self-care and healthy living. I believe in the process. It certainly worked for me and my family. With my business I help the clients and usually their families too. It's another way of teaching and helping others. Sometimes I work online from my dining room table or sometimes I go out and make group presentations. The flexible hours are perfect for me. Right now I have clients from seven different countries.

It was hard to accept that I would not be a school teacher. But I have found ways to work with kids like me outside of the school system and to help other people. I guess you could say that I've turned the things I'm good at, and that I value, into a career. It's a bit mix and match. My jobs change with the seasons but I always get a paycheck and I have time to be with my little ones. The job I dreamed about and worked toward for so many years hasn't come along, but the revised plan is working pretty well.

Looking Back
There was a real lack of resources for me in elementary and high school. Today inclusion and accommodations are expected. I think they were just a theory then. Schools could buy in to programming for disabilities or not. As for assistive technology, there was nothing. When it came to the big year-end exams, everyone else was in the gym and I would write in a separate classroom. But the separate classroom had thirty other kids in it too. It was not that helpful! People would ask my parents why they didn't send me to a special school and they would say "Why don't they come down the road and set up programs here?" That's still what they believe. They don't want to give up on this community. They want us to have the resources we need.

Today I do the same things as my parents did. I twist people's arms to come down here. I know they will love it if they come. They will see why it's great to be here. Maybe because people here didn't give up, the situation is much better for my kids than it was for me. We have more resources in the schools and in the community. We even have a pilot program for kids with autism. It is working so well that a family moved here from the city so their child could participate. Now that is something different!

When I went to university it was a big change to have an official program of supports and technology available to me. At first I had an old-fashioned computer that took up a whole kitchen table. Then I got a new light weight computer and a digital recorder. I used a lap top in lecture halls. It was great. Instead of being stuck on a word I could get the first three or four letters of a word and use autocorrect or the prediction feature to keep moving on. My last computer was very light weight and portable but it couldn't do what the portable devices can do now. Eventually I got one of those scan-and-read pens which I still keep in my purse. It comes in handy for those surprise forms and print directions. But now, when I need something spelled or read, I use my Smartphone like everyone else. The advances in technology are really something to get excited about.

It took me a while to learn to use all of my supports and not just the technology. At first I didn't know what to do with the people around me. I didn't really know what I needed and I didn't know who to ask for what. By the end of my time at university I was comfortable with a whole range of things to try when the learning system didn't fit me. Using technology and becoming comfortable with different options turned out to be really useful to me. Technology really helped me feel more independent but I also needed that support team especially to get me started. By the end of my time at university it felt like we were all working together as a team and I was helping other students with disabilities too.

I would say that at university there were courses that opened my eyes. They would be the ones in human kinetics. That was the area I was really interested in. Some of the professors in that department were great for me. The more experience people had with different ways of learning, the better it was for me. In the human kinetics department most of the people there learned hands on anyway. The students and the professors could relate to stepping away from the books, the pens and the paper. If you asked me right now what I remember from doing courses outside of kinetics (ones I was required to take to get into education) I'd have to say "not much". I'm sure those courses were great for other kinds of teachers but for me not so much.

When I think about my university years, it seems as if they were just something that I had to do to have a career as a teacher. Here you need an undergraduate degree to be eligible to take teacher training. Then you take another two years to get your Bachelor of Education degree. In those undergraduate years, I was always trying to adapt and learn in a system that wasn't suited to me. It was hard work and often frustrating but the reward was the qualification. Also, I did think about some things differently after university. Doing my degree was a kind of broadening experience. I suppose that might have come from moving out and not living with my parents too, but I needed to learn more than that. Going to university wasn't fun. It's not that I regret going, since it really changed the way I did things. Technology was definitely a big take away but it wasn't just that. If I hadn't gone through all of that struggle, where would I have learned all that I could do with some good strategies and hard work? University gave me confidence that I could get things done even when the system presents me with a whole bunch of obstacles.

Family

As important as a career is to me, my family is first and where most of my time goes. My husband and I now have three boys and at the moment they are all under six. My parents are beyond delighted and they love helping out. My husband's job involves working away six months of the year, a few weeks at a time, so it's great to have them close by. Life is always busy. Our boys love being outside and since we live in the woods it's easy to find things to do outdoors. Some days though my main job is bus driver for clubs or classes or school and daycare.

Last year we took our eldest boy out of the woods, put a polo shirt and a back-pack on him and sent him to school. It must have been quite the shock. Like his parents he doesn't find reading all that pleasurable but he likes the social side of being in school. The classroom teachers are pretty good. We seem to get the young ones starting out but they don't usually stay very long. Consistency is a bit of an issue and unsettling for my little one by times. He is a bit down these days. His best buddy had a death in his family and my son is trying to figure that out and help his friend. You know he is really bright and always on the move but he's pretty thoughtful and caring. You could call him a social butterfly.

Unlike the situation for my husband and me, our little guy has been in a literacy support program since grade primary. It's great to have the school support. He has a teacher that works with him individually and she sends work home for him too. He works both inside and outside of class with her but everything is arranged so that he doesn't miss the fun things or anything the other kids do. Last week he came home really excited with a book "to keep". It was the first book he had finished on his own. For him right now school is a good place. Here's hoping it will be for the other two as well.

I strongly believe there is a genetic connection for learning. I think all three boys are like their parents. There is no paper trail in my husband's family but I see the same signs in them as there is in my crowd. Between my family and my husband's family how could they escape? Their grandmother works for Early Childhood Intervention and every once in a while she gets out her charts and norms to keep an eye on my three. Apparently they were late talkers and none of them took to reading books without a push.

We have a house full of books and words and lots of activities and ways to learn. At home we all read together. The expectation is for them to learn and to read but we know there are different ways of reading and learning. We read audio books and we have them in the truck too, since country people do lots of travelling. We use the closed captioning feature on the TV so we can see the words. I have sticky notes all over the house with the words for various objects. We play cue card word games. I can do things at home but it's good to have someone besides me trying to get my son comfortable with print. I want my kids to able to figure out how to learn and do the things they want to do even if it's in a different way. I expect the best from my kids the way my parents did for me. Those expectations and my parents' belief in my abilities made a big difference in my life. I'm sure I would not be where I am today without that.

Looking Forward

So here I am today. I definitely don't think of myself as having a problem and I don't think of myself as a person with a disability. I feel that I am a person who knows herself well. I know the things I can do. We are all individuals and we do things differently. It's apparently not a big deal when you are not in a structured learning situation like university. I enjoy reading now that I use audio books. They are all the rage with the kids too. They are great for bedtime stories and entertainment for trips. When I get audio books at the library people say "Oh, that's cool. What a good idea. Maybe I should try that it would be great on car trips". They don't say "Why are you doing that? What's your problem?"

In life you can just do things the way you can. I might sit next to a person at a meeting and they do something one way and I do it another. To tell the truth I don't even notice anymore. I always have my Smartphone with me. It's great. You can use it for a bunch of things.

In high school I would sit there and stare trying to get my brain to work out how to spell a word. With the Smartphone I just say the word and up it pops on my screen. I can use it anywhere. Maybe it's like being colour blind. I don't notice that there is a difference anymore. As long as I have my Smartphone, I'm good to go.

My big desk top computer is great for keeping in touch with people and for working. With my on-line business I am on the computer everyday, making money and expanding my world without having to leave home. If people ask me for information, I always offer to send it to them electronically. It's an accurate copy that way and the spelling is all good without me struggling. All of those strategies have become automatic for me. I don't even think about it anymore.

I am on a literacy committee for the district. Can you believe that! Three levels of government are trying to work on a plan to improve the literacy levels in our area and I'm there. Apparently, as a group, we are significantly below the averages for the country. I listen to the oral presentations and take my notes. They circulate one or two-page summaries for the key points to everyone. I read them but I don't think most people read all the handouts. My learning disability hasn't come up. I don't talk about it much in my community. I know I used to do all that public education but I never did down here. There are people here who would think less of you if they knew. I don't want to have to deal with that. I don't want to try to explain or change people's views. I just want to be there and work on improving literacy or do my share in whatever project I am working on.

When people ask me how I'm doing I usually say "life is normal." I guess everyone's normal is different so maybe what I mean is life is pretty good and I know it could be worse. I've learned through my business to count your blessings and be grateful for every day. The day-to-day is never dull with three kids under six. I feel lucky most days to be able to be present with them as they grow especially since their dad is away a lot. I think it's important that I am here with them.

I'm excited about my online business and the possibilities it opens up for me. I am really busy but I can have a schedule that allows me to keep it all and still care for my family. I would never have that flexibility as a teacher in a school. I don't even think of looking at those job ads these days. The skating club is thriving and I can't imagine not being part of the folk festival. The courses I took to start my business emphasized the value of positive thinking and having a clear vision of where you want to go. Since setting goals and making a plan is what I have been doing for years I liked having that affirmed.

My goals haven't really changed that much. I am home living where I have always wanted to live with my husband and family. I have a career where I teach and help others. It's not quite the way I had planned but most days I think I am doing the right things and moving forward.

THE VIEW FROM OUTSIDE

The dream of becoming a teacher made it necessary for both Sophie and Alice to go to university and perform in areas where they were not naturally gifted. They arrived at university almost unaware of the reality of their learning situations. It's not easy as an adult to acquire the awareness and strategies that will allow you to succeed at university but hard work was never an issue for either of them. After the failure experiences of her first year Sophie began to examine and change her ways of dealing with academic tasks. Once she accepted the need to "deal with her learning disability" she applied her strengths and problem-solving skills to her academic work and successes followed. Alice was more reluctant to abandon her old strategies and find new ways of "working with her learning disability instead of against it". She had a long hard road in those years. At times Alice's determination seemed to work against her and block the way to better choices. Somehow time after time, she found second chances and eventually accommodations that worked for her. There were obstacles to be managed but neither Alice nor Sophie wavered or gave up on earning their Bachelor of Education degree. Seven years of formal study is a long time but never giving up had always been a big part of their success. They now had credentials plus their practical experience to offer any hiring committee that was looking for a school teacher. It looked as if the stage was set for them to reach their goal.

We only know the outline of Alice's story beyond graduation from the intermittent contact that I had with her. She had begun to experience health problems during her years in the Bachelor of Education program. Her increased environmental sensitivities added to the accommodations she required but immediately after graduation she was hired to teach in a remote northern community. It was a big step but she was excited and willing to move to take her chance. She believed that the community's enthusiasm for her student-centered teaching approaches would make the position a good match for what she needed and could offer. As time passed it became clear this was not the case. Before the end of the school year, Alice had returned to the Maritimes. She had pursued her dream to the limits of her strength but being a teacher in that classroom was not possible. It was a difficult reality to face. Alice knew she had to rest and regroup. She was not well enough to think of applying for further classroom jobs. She went back to teaching the mathematics she loved in the tutoring sessions, workshops and day camps of her past. As her stresses lessened her strength returned. Her faith community had always been an important support to Alice and a source of strength. They valued her fellowship and the contributions she made. Once again, she found a place among them to be a leader and a teacher. She also found a partner there and began building a family of her own. After a heart-breaking disappointment, she has found new dreams and plans that have taken her across the country and out of touch.

Sophie too met challenges in securing her dream job and she shows us the details of how she found a path to a set of new career options. During her last two years at university, Sophie thrived. She found the Education program suited her skills and interests very well. After graduation she was confident and ready to find herself a place back home as a school teacher. She knew her partner, her home and family were there for her. It seemed that all of the parts of her 'plan' were falling into place.

This did not turn out to be the case. When Sophie returned to her community as a qualified teacher numbers of school age students in her community were declining and teaching positions were scarce. In spite of her best efforts and many attempts she could not find a way to become the successful candidate in any of the local competitions. Hard work, determination and all of the experience and degrees she had acquired were not enough to get her that dream job. She gives us a vivid description of those stressful and frustrating years that led to her finding new career options.

Sophie developed a back-up plan to move beyond the roadblocks to her original career goal. She combined the skills and strategies she gained at university with her past successes in the community and found herself a variety of employment options. Now Sophie is outside of the confines of the classroom and teaching skills to kids and parents. She is helping others find their own remedies for a healthier, happier life. Technology has helped her to manage in the day-to-day and to widen her world without leaving home. In the process of revising her plan, she has developed new resources for her community and created a successful online business. Adjusting 'the plan' has allowed her to work and to live where she wants to be.

More than once Sophie has broken through the cycles of negativity that surrounded her. Once she accepted that her goal of teaching and helping children like her would have to be achieved in another way, she generated a wealth of good ideas and enjoys doing the work of making them happen. It is easy to admire her strength and resilience. Now that she is outside the structures of the formal education system she is more comfortable. She doesn't feel the impact of what she learned at university to call her 'disability'. The enabling strategies that she learned are now automatic and she is passing along her understanding of different ways of doing things to her children and to the community.

You might wonder if Sophie would have had a better chance of being a school teacher in another location. What if she had been willing to move? This question doesn't seem to haunt Sophie. She may have had some tough choices to make but one thing she was sure of was her desire to be part of the community where she grew up. That part of the plan was too important to give up. Her sense of place and home, the value of friendships and loving relationships were powerful enough to keep her looking for alternative ways to teach and help others.

Sophie is home, where she always wanted to be, living a busy action-packed life with her husband and three children. She found ways to use her strengths and build herself a career that allowed her to stay in her community and have meaningful work. Her determination and her ability to make a plan and see it through was a great strength but it was her ability to be flexible and creative that has allowed her to develop a multi-faceted career back home in the community that she loves. It looks like a varied and rewarding life almost exactly the way she dreamed it might be. Maybe better?

Planning, hard work and determination are clearly building blocks for success. They took both Alice and Sophie a long way toward their dreams. At the same time, their stories show us that sometimes that is not enough. Finding a good fit for their abilities as teachers in the education system turned out to be too big a challenge for them to meet. Adjusting the goals of a dream that has pulled you through many difficult times is not easy. Succeeding in the face of failures and mastering all kinds of challenges against the odds, makes it hard to know when to redirect your energies. In building their careers, both of these young women needed to be flexible and creative problem solvers as well as determined. They had to find other ways and places to express their strengths and their desire to help others. To accomplish their career dreams, they needed to reshape them for the realities and opportunities in the world around them. This is what has given them success.

10
JAY SIMPSON
University Years

The first thing I remember about coming to university was opening the door of my parents' car, stepping onto the campus and meeting someone I knew from home. She was the vice-president of the Students' Union and she looked happy to see me. I felt better immediately. I thought, "This might be a step in the right direction!"

The second thing I remember was going to the Counselling Centre and meeting the person who worked with students with disabilities. A friend from home had told me to go over there right away. Before that visit, even though I had been accepted into the university and I had received a student loan, I was still questioning if university was the place for me. After that visit, I knew there was someone in the place that I could talk to who understood and could help. I didn't have to worry about a whole bunch of special problems anymore. It relaxed me to think that I wasn't going to have to do this all alone. Walking back to the residence, I felt much more comfortable. Like everybody else, all I had to worry about was how the hell I was going to survive orientation.

Meeting those two people was critical for me. It made me feel good about being at university and I began to think that I just might succeed. I felt I had opened that door and got off to a very good start.

First Year

Coming to university meant a great deal to me. I had spent an extra year in high school to make sure I was prepared, but I still had to spend first year trying to sort out what happens at a university. This world was new to me. My mind was full of unanswered questions. What is expected? What difference does my learning disability make? Can I make it? I wasn't sure what I could expect from myself. I knew my writing skills were below most people but I didn't know how that would affect me. I didn't always understand the things going on around me. There was no one who had already gone to university that I knew well enough to help me with my questions. The university experience wasn't part of my family background. My parents were happy to see me do well and they were very encouraging, but they didn't really understand what I was doing or how I was doing it.

To get the kind of feedback and support that I knew I needed, I met every week for strategy sessions with the counsellor. I felt like she was one of the people who really understood both what I was doing and what I was trying to do. I could communicate what I was thinking and feeling. We discussed things in terms that I understood. Once we started talking about learning strategies and planning, I think about ninety per cent of our talks were about baseball. That was the way I was able to deal with what was going on.

I love baseball and I had done some coaching. I would come in and look at myself, not always objectively, but as a coach. Just as a batting average tells you how well you are hitting, I established ways of measuring how well I was doing. As a player you get the results, but as a coach it's important to know why you got them. Maybe your swing is totally off? Maybe your stance is the problem? That is how I had to learn to assess my academic performance. Each test became a kind of benchmark. We would discuss what I was doing and how I was doing it. I found those talks really significant in moving me along.

Relationships are my resources. Much about my relationship with the counsellor worked for me. She gave me the benefit of the doubt more than I would ever have given myself, especially early on when I didn't understand the expectations or the norms. She always seemed to be on my side and I knew I could count on her in a crisis.

The day that I heard from the Department of Vocational Rehabilitation that they would fund my university studies was the day I learned for sure that I could count on her to see my side of things. In our region, I was the first person with a learning disability to receive funding in a university program. The director of the department stressed that they would be monitoring my progress closely. How I performed would decide whether or not they would fund other students with learning disabilities. My counsellor saw immediately how much pressure that put on me and asked if that felt like too much of a burden for me to handle. It was added pressure, but in a way I wanted that. It meant I couldn't get complacent. I've always found it easier to do things for others. The thought that I wasn't just in this for me, and that my success could open opportunities for other people, was a reason to keep on trying even though I might feel discouraged. I couldn't just settle for getting through. But as much as I valued that pressure from outside, I think it was important that she never put that pressure on me.

One other situation where I really needed an advocate stands out. I had taken an introductory English class with a writing component. I spent a lot of time learning how to structure a paper. We had to do a short paper of five or six pages every two weeks. I learned a lot about developing an argument and presenting it in writing. It was really useful. I could see the improvement in my written work, but that was with a spell check, grammar check and a friend to type for me. The grammar and spelling section of the course was done on our own using a computerized program. I could not master it. After hours of working on that computer program, I scored a worse mark on the post-test than I had on the pre-test. The counsellor helped me negotiate a release from the grammar section. Otherwise my English mark would have been ruined.

There were several times that year when I needed help. The incident that I'll never forget happened during my final exams. The professor didn't show up as we had arranged and he hadn't made any provisions for me to write an accommodated exam. Nothing had been set up as he had promised. I was really in a panic situation. I went to the counsellor. She calmed me down and got me through that day. We talked about options when I couldn't see any. She reminded me that I had written exams all through high school without accommodation. She called the professor. There had been a family emergency and I had been forgotten. We worked out a back-up plan. I wrote the exam without accommodation, but I could negotiate the mark afterwards and have an oral exam if I wished. It worked out, but I'll never forget how that felt. I would not have wanted to be in that situation without an ally.

When people would be difficult about accommodations, or when they wouldn't follow through with the arrangements we had made, the counsellor would get angry. She got angry when I couldn't. It made me feel good and I'd tell myself I'd better work on a solution to calm her down. I just couldn't deal with getting angry myself. I say that more in retrospect than from my sense of things at the time. Even now I find it very difficult to get angry at people. It just doesn't do me any good. I usually feel it's probably my fault that things have gone wrong. The counsellor expressed those feelings for me and showed me ways of getting around the problems. I started to understand how to develop working relationships with the professors. In the end, I learned a lot about negotiation skills and different ways to accommodate my learning style at university. These were really important skills to build on over the next few years.

Meanwhile, back in residence, a lot of people helped me with the details of being social. They gave me lots of very direct information about the do's and don'ts of residence life. I guess it was either because they cared, or because they didn't like to be mean and wanted me to have friends. It made my life easier. They pretty much covered all of the expectations right down to "Don't eat with your mouth open!" and "Don't invade people's space!" I learned how to live with forty guys.

Living with forty people who were students made a big difference for me. I got to see a whole lot of right things and wrong things to do. With partying I was able to set limits, because I knew why I was at university. At home I had always been involved in alcohol awareness activities. I felt that I had a side of myself that could easily become addicted to alcohol, so I decided when I was young that I didn't want to use it. I had seen too many people's lives being destroyed because they couldn't set those limits. To go to a bar, listen to loud music, get loaded while talking about getting loaded was never my idea of fun. It turned out to be a big advantage to have figured this out before I arrived at university.

Socially I am pretty shy, so residence was great for me. It was a ready-made group. I like to talk and I like debating. There were all kinds of other people who liked those things and were good at them too. When you live in a university residence you're not such an odd ball because you're interested in politics. There were fifty other people interested too. Even at two o'clock in the morning, there was always a room with a discussion going on. I enjoyed the company and there were a whole bunch of casual learning experiences that I could tap into. I was able to watch and learn and listen, as well as make some good friends. It suited my learning style perfectly. I count residence life as one of the highlights of my first year.

Academically a major turning point for me was my political science course. My professor knew about learning disabilities and he knew students with learning disabilities who had done well at university. For the first exam, the professor had me write in the class with everyone else and then he asked me to record my answers to the exam on an audiotape. It was the first time that I had used a dictaphone to present my ideas without having to write them down. What a difference! I could see how my writing skills affected what I could tell people. It was such an important moment for me that I'm sure I could dictate that paper word for word today.

After doing that exam on tape I saw that it was not only all right to work orally, but that doing oral exams was a way that I could excel. I saw that there were professors who would allow me to work that way, and people in the learning center who would help me figure out how to do it. I started learning how to use the dictaphone effectively. I made friends with the woman who did the dictatyping. I knew that I had found a strategy that would make a huge difference in helping me deal with my writing problems and allowing me to show what I knew.

In that political science course, I asked questions in class and joined in the discussion. I sat in the same row as the best students. They were always willing to lend me their notes and to discuss things with me. I had a lot of respect for them as people and as students. I tried to model a lot of what they did. To be one of them was really important to me. When it came time for the Christmas exam, I got the dictaphone and 'wrote' the exam. I scored 80 per cent, an A grade. Those people in my row knew as much as I did and with an eighty I was able to be one of them. I was in the right place. All of a sudden it was real to me! I was at university.

I did a lot of right things that first year, even though they weren't exactly conscious strategies. I was diligent. I never missed a class and I took every mini-course the university offered: how to study, how to use the library, how to write papers. You name it, I was there. I had two really good friends from home who were in first year with me. They weren't always in my classes but I always knew that I could count on them to help with studying, a paper, or just about anything. I asked questions in classes and in the professors' office hours. I was visible. The professors could see that I was knowledgeable and that I was interested. That interest was my currency. I really wanted to be at university and no one doubted that.

It was the friendships I brought with me and the friendships I developed that made that first year possible. I felt as if I was getting anchors down so that I could stay. All of those people, students and professors, my dictatypist and my counsellor, were my resources. They were all a critical part of the whole process for me. There were high points and low points that first year. There were moments of panic, but once I found the right people, I felt that I had all the resources necessary to succeed like anyone else.

Year Two

Sounds great so far doesn't it? But good first innings don't mean that there's nothing left to be done. Second year was really rough. Even though I started full of confidence, second year turned out to be one of those critical times when things could have gone one way or another. Sometimes I wasn't sure that I could stay. I had decided to do an honours degree in political science, even though I knew it was a tough degree to obtain. I wanted to write a thesis and succeed at the toughest challenge. I wanted to be like those people who were my peers in political science and my first year marks were good enough to get me into the program.

It seemed that in first year everything just fell into place. Second year, I couldn't seem to get into the right courses. I have never shifted so many classes. I hate shifting classes. I like to be there right from the first day of the course. I changed from history to english. I changed economics professors three times trying to get the right professor for me. I had trouble adjusting to the lecture styles of my political science professors. I signed on for an introductory psychology course in case I wanted to take an education degree later. My counsellor had warned me about the difficulties of both economics and psychology for a person with my learning pattern but I liked the topics and they fit my degree plan. I even had a background in economics from high school. I thought that would be enough to get me through. I didn't believe that my learning disability would limit me seriously. My first year had given me confidence.

As it turned out, I really struggled with economics. I just couldn't do the mathematics. I would meet with the professor for extra help. He would go over the graphs with me. We would have a great discussion about the concepts from class or the economy of Cape Breton, but I still couldn't do the math or deal with the graphs.

I struggled with psychology too. I couldn't keep the details and the terms straight. It must have taken me all year to try to understand what cognitive meant. I just couldn't get my mind around it. I was interested in the course and I always had lots of questions. I felt I understood a lot of the ideas and their significance, but passing the tests was another matter. Both of these courses were at the introductory level and it hurt my self-confidence to see those poor marks. I spent a lot of time and worry just trying to pass. Fortunately I knew some senior students with learning disabilities. Their experiences were similar to mine and that helped me to accept what was happening even though I couldn't change it.

Adding to my disappointment, I didn't do that well in my political science courses either. I think I learned the difference between partisan politics and political science the hard way. It also turned out that I had a lot more to learn about being a student. In spite of all of the set-backs, I was able to maintain an average above seventy that allowed me to stay in the honours program, but it was a pressure year for sure!

What changed? Course selection was part of the problem, but second year presented a new set of demands and I had a whole new set of skills and strategies to learn. I couldn't just remember everything I heard and be a top student. Even though I had a strong background in political science, I wasn't familiar with everything that was going on in class anymore. All of the information wasn't presented in class either. I actually had to learn how to take in written information and turn it around into useable knowledge. This was new for me. I had never had to rely on print before and I'm not sure that I was really aware of that fact. Reading was slow and tiring, but I thought that I just didn't particularly enjoy reading. I didn't realize that reading was a problem for me.

It became clear that I had to develop some new strategies for getting all of the important information. Because of my reading speed, I had to figure out what was critical to read and what I could leave out. This was easier to figure out in political science than in my other courses because I could ask the good students who were working at my level. In psychology, social referencing was harder and I found it harder to understand the readings. Suggestions from the good students didn't help since I wasn't dealing with the material at their level. I didn't know what to make of the suggestions from the students who, like me, were just getting by. I knew I had to pick different strategies than they did because I had different problems and I wanted better results. I couldn't read everything and I wasn't comfortable asking the professors how to cut down the reading. It was trial and error.

I tried to find people who would discuss readings and classes with me. Sometimes I would get people to read to me while they did their own work. I much preferred these methods of getting the information, but it's not always possible to find study groups and keep them going. People get busy and I can't seem to follow a routine. My friends were like that too. It was hit and miss, but it worked out pretty well for some lively discussion, especially the night before a test.

Perhaps my biggest accomplishment in second year was learning how to access the information that was available in the library. I thought that I had learned how to use the library and write a paper in first year. I soon realized that those early papers had been short. Since I understood the format and how to develop the argument, I could sit with the dictaphone and rip off six pages on a topic without too much research. Now I had to find and check multiple sources. I had to learn to gather and organize written material. I had big trouble with quotes, especially getting them down straight, and figuring out how to build them into my paper. It was very frustrating and seemed to take a huge amount of time.

I got to know the ladies in the library really well and they were very good to me. They taught me the system, including the tricks and some very valuable shortcuts. I caught onto the technology right away, but there were all kinds of simple, basic things about indices, periodicals and documents that I just didn't know how to use. I didn't know that you could check at the end of an article for all of the references that the author had used. I had always just ignored that part. The librarians made me feel comfortable enough to ask and they would help me find things when I couldn't manage. They gave me extra time for the reserve readings. They were even willing to ignore the fact that I usually couldn't find my card. They were great! I didn't realize at that point how well those hours would pay off during the rest of my time at university.

I finished the year with some important new skills, and a much better understanding of what I was good at and what I wasn't. If I had it to do over again, I would probably do the same thing. I think that year I had to test the waters and find out what I could do, even if it meant struggling. As it turned out, I didn't really need economics for my program but I did need psychology in order to go on to become a teacher. My marks weren't the best, but I scraped through in the tough courses and I did well enough in the others to stay in the honours program.

It was fortunate that I could gloss over a year that was bad for courses with a good year socially. I had become involved in campus activities and made some really good friends. When I got my marks I was upset, but I could deal with it because part of my life was going well and I hadn't done any serious damage to my record. Academically the whole year had been a struggle. Not once could I lift my head and walk away from my desk feeling that everything was under control. It was worth the struggle because after that year academics kind of fell into place for me.

Summer in the City

The summer between second and third year was one more season of finding out what I could do and what I couldn't. I decided to go to Ottawa to look for work. I liked the idea of going off on my own. I had an aunt I could stay with and I knew some students from Ottawa. I got a job stock-taking for the government. Every day at work I was confronted with the fact that I was reversing all the numbers and inverting things. Not only that, I was the slowest person there. It was like a flash of bright light. I suddenly realized, "I have a learning disability." It had not really become clear to me until that day at work. It was just all of a sudden, WHACK! That job made my learning disability real to me.

I know it seems impossible, but even though I had talked about being learning disabled and used the label, it still wasn't part of me until that moment. Even though I had gone through the whole process of identifying myself at university, taking tests and being assessed by professionals, all of that, I just hadn't accepted that it was so basic and so pervasive. I used to think that I read well. Maybe I was a bit slow at it, but I understood things. My problem was just that I couldn't write. I saw writing as my only real problem. Then, when I got to use some technology like the dictaphone, it masked my inability to write. I still said that I wasn't a good writer, but it was pretty painless to sit with a scribe or a recorder and do my exams. The papers were still pain and struggle, even with the dictaphone, but when I got them typed they looked really good. I couldn't believe that I had written them. They weren't the papers of a person who couldn't write.

It was a very tough summer. I realized a lot of things. That environment was not where I belonged. I wasn't good at my job. I didn't have the friendship and support that I was used to. I wasn't accustomed to the way people lived in Ontario. Nothing was easy for me, not even getting around the city. I really missed being involved with baseball and I realized that coaching a team was important to my self-esteem. All you have to do as a coach is walk onto the field and you're significant to the twelve people on the team. The things you have to do as a coach don't seem difficult to me, and you can make people feel better with the least little gesture, or just by listening to them. I really missed being a coach.

Living through that summer wasn't pleasant, but I'm glad I went away. I gained some experience and confidence. I came home knowing that there was no future for me in being a stock boy. I was going to have to do something that involved thinking and reasoning. I had to play to my strengths and try to minimize the impact of my weaknesses. I was determined to do well academically and to learn more about being a good baseball coach.

Third Year
Of all the years I spent at university, I think this was the most

enjoyable. I made a lot of right choices and I did play to my strengths. I went back to political science, english and history. I could use my intuition in those subjects and do well. I had a feeling for the material, and I knew how to make a good argument and presentation. I was able to prove that to my professors early in the year. Then it was easy to continue to do well and get exam accommodation. I was always in class and I always participated in discussions. If my papers were a bit late, the professors didn't seem to mind. They knew I was interested and that I was working.

My political science professor in first year had recommended that, if I was serious about political science, it was important for me to get information from professors with different academic frameworks and different teaching styles. In a small university, it is tempting for students with a disability to stick with professors who will accommodate their learning style and who have given them good marks in the past. In second year I had found the adjustment to new professors difficult, but by third year it added variety and interest to my courses. I think it also made me a better learner. By the time I finished university, I had managed to succeed even with professors who were intimidating. I learned to use the fear factor instead of letting it defeat me.

Overall, I found that I had the most trouble with professors who were spontaneous and entertaining, but were all over the map in the lectures. Often these professors are very popular with students, but I need more structure. I knew I wasn't playing it safe by trying new professors, but I also knew that I was really interested in political science. In third year I lucked out. My professors were really inspiring that year. Even though their styles were quite different, they all presented material in an organized and structured way that made it easy for me to learn. I was comfortable enough to speak to them after class if there was something I didn't understand.

I was lucky with my friends too. I met some wonderful people in the campus activities I joined. Extra-curricular activities were my chance to be good at something and meet people at the same time. The debating society is a great example. My oral skills are strong and in debating I never had to write. I could demonstrate and strengthen my ability to develop arguments in a logical step-by-step fashion. All of this, and I was meeting other students and touring the province.

In some activities I was a club member. Other times I took on a leadership role. It made me feel good to be a president or a vice-president. Sometimes I was able to work with the professors on projects too. Knowing all of these people outside of the classroom just seemed to feed into my success. It made me feel that I had built up some currency and it made it easier for me to ask for help with courses. There were a few people that I just clicked with. Often they were in some of my classes too. They seemed to be good academically as well as really involved in campus life. This made my year really enjoyable and all these people were excellent resources for my studies.

There was a friend from student government in my history class. He wasn't very good at history, but I was. He was really popular and could borrow good notes easily. He found it really helpful to talk over the readings and the class material. We became study buddies. He got the notes and I did the talking. We both felt we were contributing so it was an ideal arrangement for both of us. That year I also had two excellent note takers. Between those two types of arrangements, I was able to have good sets of notes for all of my courses.

Sometimes it's hard to find note takers who take the kind of notes that fit your study needs. Sometimes you can't rely on good note takers to be at every class. I did have a problem with one of my note takers, but not the usual kind of problem. This person was the best note taker I have ever had. He was a friend from home. We had taken some of our classes together ever since first year and he had always done notes for me. He was a very good student with excellent marks. Now I was doing just as well as he was and that had never been the case before. Sometimes I even got a better mark than he did, and here he was doing notes for me! For the first time, I felt that he resented the note taking arrangement. Not that he wanted to see me doing poorly, but I felt that he resented the fact that I was able to compete with him and win. I know that I am competitive, but he feigns not being competitive at all. I felt a difference. He denied it. We still joke about this and he continues to be a great support and friend to me, but we are not in the same classes anymore.

Personal things like that seemed to be the critical part of third year for me. I was figuring out who I was and what I was trying to do at university. I had come back from the summer in Ottawa with a new sense of my learning disability. I was aware of my weaknesses more than ever before, but I was doing better academically than I had ever done before. I found it very awkward having to deal with how other people felt about my disability, especially in the face of my academic success. Some people made it plain that they thought it was all a game and some days I wanted to believe them. I had always felt that I had two things going for me. I was a good person and I knew myself. That year I was confused.

Even though most people would tell you that I'm very outgoing and talkative, I am really shy and don't want to be hurt. Before I came to university, most of the people I knew I had grown up with. Now my circle of friends had grown. I spoke to all kinds of people, but I wasn't sure where I belonged or how to read these people or events. Sometimes it was exciting and enjoyable, but I wasn't always sure where people were coming from or what they intended by some of their comments.

I don't know if there are some people who can just automatically understand these things, but for me it was a skill that I had to acquire. It took me a while and some more sessions with my counsellor. I would bring the stories of all of these people and situations into the office, and we would discuss them. That year I learned how to take a compliment, how to deal with people who weren't very nice, how to confront people and how to let them know what you feel. I began to see that sometimes it is better not to just ignore things and let them roll off. It was an important learning experience for me.

In third year everything was there for me. Both my social and academic life were in balance. My marks had improved. I had learned that I was capable of good academic work. That question was answered. Now there were new ones. What was my potential? Where were my limits? How could I be as good as I could be?

Summer on the Sandlot

I went home for the summer and talked Russell (the best coach in the league) into teaching me how to coach. I realized that I had only been a nursemaid up to that point. I had gone into managing and coaching baseball because as much as I knew and loved the game, I just couldn't execute the plays. I didn't have the physical skills. Russell appreciated my dedication and the summers I had already put in, so he agreed to teach me. From that point on I really started to improve. Russell taught me the game and what it meant to play it well. I learned organizational skills. I learned how to break down a big task (like organizing a tournament) into the necessary parts, prioritize the list and get everything done.

Russell's philosophy was that if you work hard, you get rewards. He maintained that was the same kind of effort that you had to put into life. That summer I finally made that connection. I believed in hard work because I had watched my dad do it all of his life. As I got older I said, "What kind of reward did he get? He got two bad knees and a bad pension. Some reward!" With Russell, when we put the time in, we always won.

That season we played thirty games. The kids worked hard. We got uniforms. We all did what we were supposed to do. We had the best team in the whole province and it was all because we were willing to do what it took to make it happen. That's the attitude that I took, coming into fourth year with my thesis looming. "If I get organized, put in the time and effort and do what it takes to make it happen, I will be successful."

Fourth Year and Graduation

Fourth year turned out to be the most severe test yet of my strength and determination. I guess you get your mettle tested in the fire and I think I spent the whole year in the fire. By the end of the year I knew that if I could survive this, I could survive anything.

I thought I had a good plan for the year and I got an early start. I knew I needed to have good marks for any of the things I wanted to do next. Law school, education and social work were the programs I was considering. I needed the courses that would get me there. Once again I decided to play to my learning strengths. I knew some things I wanted to do better, but I felt I knew enough about my learning strategies to make good choices and to see them through. I knew the paper I wanted to write for my thesis and I found an advisor who knew the area. I set things up before classes began. I had an impressive list of extra-curricular commitments that would be lots of fun and would look great on my resume. I decided to move out of residence on campus into a house with some friends. I was really looking forward to my graduating year.

I had been talking with my counsellor about time management since first year. This had always been a problem. I specialized in improvising last minute solutions to get me out of trouble. I was determined to do better that year. But it seems that with time management I can't be consistent. I've always just used the techniques when things get rough, like shifting into high gear and getting through the rough patch. As long as the road is flat and things are going smoothly, I ignore all the things that I know about time management. I feel they tie me down too much. They don't let me do the things I'm good at. Being creative, spontaneous and intuitively sorting out problems is what I do best. Where would using a day planner get me? I'd only lose it. I forget to write things down. I put them under the wrong day. I don't really trust what I write down anyway. Are you convinced?

I discussed plan after plan with my counsellor, but I wasn't really listening or doing any of it. The more I planned, the worse it got. Now I think that I was focusing on time management to avoid what was really going on. It was fear. I was afraid that I had taken on too much and I couldn't admit that. I told myself it would just be a question of getting into the right mind set when it came time to meet my deadlines.

I think of myself as working well under pressure. I knew students who wrote their papers weeks in advance so that they could go back, edit and polish what they had written. I know these are important things to do, but I could never do it. I'd have all the research done. I would happily put in my time at the library. I could explore the topic and make the connections, but I could not force myself to sit down and write the paper. I would find a million other things to do. Anything but sit down and write that paper! Then, when the moment comes that there can be no more excuses and no more extensions, I sit down and produce. Sometimes this really works well, but if I haven't fully understood the topic and processed it internally, I'm sunk. I feel I need pressure to make me sit down and write. Writing is still very frustrating for me, even with a dictaphone. As the pressure mounted, things weren't working as I had planned. A certain amount of pressure may be helpful, but the amount of pressure I got myself into in fourth year was not healthy.

My sociology course had written assignments due every two weeks. We had to describe and analyze different situations, drawing on our own experience and the sociological perspectives we were studying. I enjoyed the course and it taught me new ways of looking at the world. In the end it gave me a real sense that I could write a report that other people could understand and appreciate. Later on this turned out to be a valuable skill, but at the time it was a trial, especially with my thesis waiting for me.

I was also having some serious problems with reading. My seminar course in political science was taught by my thesis supervisor. The course had much more reading, and more difficult reading, than I had ever faced before. Short papers were required on the readings. All of a sudden reading became a big problem for me. I had never liked reading and I had never done a lot of reading for my courses. When I did read I could understand, except perhaps in psychology. That was not the case this time. In my seminar course I couldn't get through all of the material. Worse than that, I couldn't seem to see beyond the surface and make the underlying links as I had always been able to do.

I just couldn't do it. I had people reading for me, since the material wasn't available on audiotape, but it was too time consuming. There was no way that I could put in the time necessary and do all of the other things I needed to do. Everyone found the reading load heavy and part way through the term, the professor did reduce the reading requirements. I made a special arrangement that allowed me to do the readings for the seminar session, but hand my paper in a day later. The class discussion helped me get the material under control and I was able to survive.

Meanwhile, I was doing just about everything going with the Students' Union. I wasn't balancing the demands of the social and academic sides of my life. The academic demands were much more than I had anticipated. I said I didn't care. I said these commitments are really important to me. If I can come out of university with a 70 average, having done all these things, that was better than a higher average. In retrospect I'd choose a better average, but at the time I knew that was where I made my close friends, and that was what I wanted. More than that, those projects and activities reassured me that what I did in classes wasn't the whole picture. The skills that I had developed could be carried out into the world after university. They were transferable. This was proof that I could deal with what came after.

As the year went on, I became more and more worried about what would come after university. Other students were applying to graduate school or writing the law school exams. They were getting their lives in order and opening up options for the next year. I was overwhelmed as it was. I find university calendars and program descriptions to be impossible reading. I just didn't know how I could cope with filling in applications and lining up references. I also wanted to write the standardized test for admission to law school. I not only had to apply and practice for the test like everyone else, but I had to make special arrangements for testing accommodations as well. Things were piling up.

It is hard for me to convey just how difficult I find forms and paperwork. That's when I feel the most vulnerable. I always have to ask somebody to help me. Application forms are all different. They have different formats and different categories. They require a detailed description of who you are and what you have accomplished that all has to fit into those categories. You have to get organized to get references and documents in plenty of time. I can't use a dictaphone or a computer for a form. I can't type it up and expect anyone to be able to read it. I have to find someone who has the time available to sit down with me and fill in the forms. There must have been a million post-it notes stuck everywhere around my room to remind me to do each of these steps, but I wouldn't do it. I just wouldn't. I always put it off. I never did get around to completing most of my application forms, although I did write an accommodated version of the law school exams.

To add to my dilemmas, my living arrangements hadn't worked out. I always get tripped up in the details of things and living off-campus was no exception. I couldn't remember all the things to do. Did you remember to iron your pants? Did you buy food for supper? Did you do your share of the chores? What was your share of the chores? Did you lock the door? Did you turn off the stove? It felt like there were a million details to remember and that's when I start losing control. I can't focus on what I'm trying to do. It was a bad situation and it was not a happy house. I have never tried an arrangement like that again. Fortunately, I had one really good friend there and that made all the difference in the world. It got me through.

In some respects, I felt that details were my downfall throughout that year. In my thesis it was a problem, too. I could discuss the theories and the big picture, but the details of the topic were beyond me. I'm good at reading into information and analyzing the implications. I'm a good original thinker. I can draw from different types of information and perspectives, across courses and across disciplines, but when it comes to straightforward description of technical details and facts I can't manage well at all. I'm not saying I don't think details are important. It's just that I can't handle them. I think this is what annoys me the most about myself. I understand a lot about many subjects, but I can understand and discuss them only to a certain point.

For example, I could talk to you about the middle ages. I studied it years ago. I have retained a lot of the information far better than many of the people in my class. If I were to sit around and talk with experts on the middle ages, either while I was taking the class or now, I couldn't get beyond a certain depth within the material, because I cannot master the language and the details. This is my limitation. If you can't remember the names, the dates or the countries in question and you mix up the fine detail, it takes away from your power to support an argument. I can't get deep down and use the language or 'talk the talk' the way other people can. For better or worse, that's just the way I am and there's not a lot I can do about it.

As for my thesis, my supervisor was great. He was patient and helpful. We never fought once the whole time, even though my limitations were showing. Deadlines came and went. I was bogged down and couldn't get things written. One problem was that I didn't really understand the approach he wanted me to take to my topic which dealt with funding for students. In the end we compromised. I did one chapter on his issues and then set off on my own. I think in many ways I just wore him down. There were lots of other projects for him to look at and time was growing so short that there seemed no other option but to let me try my way.

I knew I had things to say and ways of getting the information that I needed. When I write that way, I am much more effective and efficient. I needed to be since the pressure was really on. One of my other political science professors and a friend from home helped me set up some critical interviews. I talked to the premier of the province, the president of the university and the student member of the provincial higher education committee. I spent the day with one of the men who had written a major work in the area. I bought his book later on, but I have to admit that I only read the parts I needed for quotation and documentation. I did three months of work in two and tried to keep everything else going as well. I don't think I have ever been more stressed in my whole, entire life. I will never forget the final month of that school year. Many times I thought everything was going to fall apart, but I did it. I wrote a thesis!

This project was a good experience in the sense that I learned a great deal. I came away with a new understanding of the discipline of political science, what it could do and what I could do. I can't answer every question, no matter how bright I am. Most important was that I finished and my thesis was accepted. Each year, only a handful of people in political science can say that. My thesis supervisor told me that my thesis was the worst written and the worst organized of all the efforts that year, but it was also the most thoughtful and the best researched. I know it was far from perfect, but for me it was still a huge accomplishment. I am dyslexic and yet I wrote a thesis. That thought has been a wonderful comfort whenever I have had to face a challenge.

But wait, that wasn't the end of fourth year yet. It may have been my greatest moment, but there was still work to be done. I remember vividly the moment when I faced the fact that I might not be able to finish all of the year's work and graduate with my class. I had submitted my thesis and written my exams, but to do that I had let other papers go unfinished. Time was running out. Nobody could extend a deadline past graduation day and I desperately wanted to walk across the stage with my class. I was exhausted. I felt that I had already done all of the impossible things that I could do. The library had closed and I was still a paper short.

I just freaked. I think my heart must have been beating about 160 times a minute. I thought it was all awash. My friend said to me, "Well Jay, you've come this far. You can either lie down and die, or you can get up and do something." So I got up and did something. My friend stood by me. I called one of my professors for some books and articles. I lined up another friend who was able to scribe for me with the computer. I did the best I could with the time remaining. It wasn't my best paper ever, but it met the requirements and it gave me a chance to graduate.

In the end I earned an honours degree in political science and I did it right on schedule. It had always been important to me to keep up with the other people in my program. I never wanted to take a course reduction no matter how hectic things were. I wanted to do everything the same way as everybody else. I felt that a course reduction would have cheapened my accomplishment and hurt my self-esteem. Right from the day I started, people were questioning my ability to qualify for a degree. I soon realized that I had to have oral exams, but I didn't want any more accommodation than was absolutely necessary. I felt I could defend the special exams and the use of the dictaphone, but not fewer courses.

A reduced course load might have been the right thing for me to do, but people had always looked at me with that little bit of lack of respect. I couldn't accept that anymore. I had grown beyond that and I wanted to prove it to people. By writing a thesis and graduating with an honours degree with my class, I felt that I had earned respect.

Looking Back

For a long while I've been thinking about what I would do differently. I find it a difficult question because I think that a lot of the things that you do are the right things for the time. I think what I did as a student was basically good, so I would maintain the core of my plan: attending class, asking questions and speaking out, talking to professors, arranging for the accommodations I needed, using the dictaphone and talking books, finding good study people to work with and good note takers.

In retrospect, I do wish I had been more organized and more

independent in turning out my written work. I know my marks suffered for being so adamant about refusing to do a reduced course load. Informally, I did have a reduced course load. Like many students, there was one course I neglected every year. The price I paid was a mark about ten per cent below the others, but I still think it was worth it to me.

The strategy of speaking out in class annoyed some of my fellow students. Some of them said that I monopolized time in class. Some people thought that I was a show off and a know-it-all. For the most part the professors didn't seem to mind me speaking up and asking questions. Often there weren't many students who actively engaged in class. Sometimes I knew that I was making some of the other students angry, but I felt I had no other choice. In first year when some of the professors saw my handwritten tests they said, "Obviously, this isn't what you know about this subject." How would they have known that if I hadn't spoken up in class?

A friend of mine who graduated the top student in the university told me that he never spoke up in class because he was afraid to make a mistake. I was afraid to say something stupid, too, just like everyone else, but not saying anything at all was the stupidest thing that I could do. I had to talk because it allowed me to sell people on how smart I was. It was a way of proving that I was interested in the course and that I was covering the reading. It showed that I was there every single day. I felt that talking would get me my accommodation. I'd hear other students with disabilities discussing how difficult it was to get accommodation from professors. I didn't have that much difficulty. Perhaps in five of the twenty-five or thirty courses that I took at university there was a problem. I think that was because I talked up.

More than that, asking questions is how I know that I'm learning. If I just sit there passively taking in information, I'm not getting anything from it. When the professor says something and I can't make any sense of it, I ask. Sometimes I'm missing a little chunk of what has gone on in the classroom, or sometimes I've made a really good point. I try to take the information through the whole process of the developing argument in my head. I'm always looking for the structure in the information. I try to make links with other things that I know. I take the material and make it my own. Then I engage the professor to see if what I'm thinking is right. Every day in class I get a little piece of the puzzle that is the course.

This strategy works as a security blanket too. The night before the test, when everyone else is trying to figure out if they've understood the material, I know because I've asked those questions all the way through the term and had my ideas confirmed by the professor. At the same time, there is no denying that I did pay a price with the other students for that strategy. But that's where the social side came in. I was part of residence life. I was in clubs and activities. The other students got to know me as a person. Then I felt I could explain about my learning disability and why I had to learn like that. Most of them became much more accepting after we had talked about my learning style.

Right from the start I think that I did a lot of the right things, but I didn't know why I was doing them. I was just following my instincts. Later on, when I was more aware of strategies that worked, I couldn't always get control over what I was doing. I think I followed a good plan to the best of my ability. I used a lot of good strategies, but I knew I was doing other things wrong and I just couldn't do anything about it. Sometimes you're just not ready or able to do what even you feel is necessary to succeed. It's the same with all of the things that you learn from listening to the stories your parents tell. You manage to use some of them and avoid problems. Other times you have to test the waters yourself. Sometimes it means making mistakes. I was fortunate enough to be able to gloss over my mistakes and get through anyway. I don't believe there is one master plan that you can sit down and follow through. That never worked for me. I think it was flexibility and determination that made my plans work.

It seems to me that the students with learning disabilities who succeed are the ones whose approach is global. They draw from both the social and academic sides of being a student to balance and complement their learning style. They are not succeeding with only one simple strategy. It's more complex than that. I don't believe there is one single strategy change that will make all the difference. There may be one factor that will make a big difference, as the dictaphone did for me, but there is no simple solution to handling a learning disability. Having a dictaphone and using taped texts won't solve every problem. If you have just one or two strategies, what happens when something goes wrong? You need to have other resources or techniques to meet the new challenges and get you through. If you don't have other options to fall back on, and you haven't placed yourself broadly in the community among people you like and trust, coping may be almost impossible.

In all honesty, I probably wouldn't change anything about my time at university, because I think that what I did was what I had to do for that time in my life. I'd keep the good and the bad. Those were the things I needed to learn and the best way I could do it at the time. In the end I came away with a degree, a real sense of accomplishment and an interest in doing further studies. I think that makes my time at university a success.

Being Learning Disabled

I was late being identified as a person with a learning disability. I didn't have a diagnosis or a label until I got into grade eight or nine. Before that I was just in what they called special reading. The term learning disability was never used in my school. Even once people outside school started using the term with reference to me, I didn't really know what it meant.

As far as I'm concerned, I was one of those students who went through the system invisible. The knocks you get going through school that way are difficult to handle. The way people treat you and act toward you, because you are different, affects your growing up. Where I lived, I was very different in a lot of ways. I didn't know what to make of how I was treated. You don't know if it's normal, or if it's right. I didn't know what to expect, or what to accept. Was I asking for special favours? Was I using my differences as a crutch? I didn't know what was a crutch and what was fair treatment. People will tell you that you are just trying to get out of work, but I was just trying to get by.

It was very important to be told that I was learning disabled. It was a relief. It said that there was something wrong with me that wasn't my fault. It explained away a lot of things. It helped me find my strengths and learn how to use them. Now, with the diagnosis that I have, I can show people that just because you can't write, it doesn't mean you can't understand or be very skilled at doing other things. That's the compensation, but it doesn't mean that it's easy to disclose your label, or talk about your differences.

For years I have been trying to sort out what part of my behaviour is my nature and what part is my learning disability? I am dyslexic. What does that mean for me? It is part of who I am and to deny that is to deny reality. One of my friends said that my learning disability shouldn't define me. I have always agreed with that, but at the same time to say that it doesn't affect you is to lie. If you are lying to yourself all the time, it just makes things a whole lot worse. Being learning disabled isn't the only thing about you, but it is one of the things about you. In certain situations, it could be the key thing about you. I certainly don't want to be a telephone operator and have to deal with 911 calls. With my ability to reverse numbers, you know that just wouldn't be a good situation.

There are situations where I feel very confident in my ability and my knowledge. Coaching minor ball would be a good example, or working on disability issues. I completed a research project on entrepreneurial training for young people with disabilities. I feel confident about the work I did and the report I have written. I know that I have a lot of strengths as well as a disability, but there are still many times and situations where I feel limited by my dyslexia.

I always have to ask myself what's real and what's not. I'm never sure. Am I in the right? Or am I in the wrong? For example, someone may call me stupid for forgetting to lock the door to the house. I have forgotten to do simple things like that so many times that I couldn't honestly say whether I did or not. It's just not the kind of thing I can remember. Someone else may have been at fault, but I don't know. At the office the other day, I took the blame for a mix up that hadn't even happened. In most things I'll make my point, but I won't push it. I'll try to find a way around a problem or a conflict rather than standing and fighting. With the level of uncertainty that I carry it's not easy to push a point, even when I feel that I am being treated unfairly.

Moments of feeling completely on top of things and in control are very fleeting for me. It's more like having a handful of strings. It's not long before one of them slips away or gets tangled up. I think that sense of control is what gives a person a feeling of power. Even in those fleeting moments when I sense that I have a position of power, I don't want to use it. I was pounded, beaten up and torn around in my community by people who had power. I remember what that felt like. I always put myself in the other person's shoes and try to find a way around obstacles rather than powering through.

Getting myself and my day organized is really hard for me. I am creative and a good spontaneous problem solver, but I've had to be. I know that it's important to manage my time to make things work smoothly, but even today I am not really effective with time management strategies. They work for a certain amount of time and then they lose their structure. Now I use a day planner, but I still don't look at it unless I know that it is going to be a particularly hectic week. I write everything in there and every morning on my busy weeks I will start the day by looking at it. If something changes and someone has forgotten to tell me, I get unnerved. I start questioning my day planner and my ability to cope. It's frustrating. Sometimes it's just easier to drift along on the presumption that the important things will come to my notice.

Some people with dyslexia are much more self-reliant than I am, especially as far as writing is concerned. I always question whether I could have done more to improve my skills with print. If I had those skills at a higher level, I would have much more independence. As it is, every time I have to fill out a form, I have to ask someone to help me. Then I have to think about what I can give them in return for doing me this favour. Sometimes it's a monetary return. Most times, it's something else. I used to get typing done by loaning out my computer to students in exchange for their typing services. Returning a favour is an essential part of my philosophy.

There are times when you just can't get around your problems with writing no matter how creative you are about exchanging skills and managing situations. Sometimes you have to take a phone message because nobody else is there. You can't always use the bank machine. Sometimes you have to go to a teller. Sometimes your note taker doesn't show up. Sometimes everyone is too busy to help you out with a form or a report. Being dyslexic leaves me with a sense of having to rely on people's good will much of the time. I don't want to burn bridges with people no matter what. People can sometimes be really difficult with me, but I realize that I might have to come back to them when I need help or an accommodation. If I make an enemy, then that's one less place I can go.

Having said all of that, I have to point out that, in a weird way, being learning disabled is what has made me special. For all of the things that I sometimes felt that it took away, it also provided opportunities to do things that I value. There are a lot of bright people out there. There are people that I went to school with who have much more on the go than I do, but haven't had the opportunities that I've had to participate in university activities and community projects. I stood out. I got to know my professors and the staff at the university. I worked closely with other students. I had to.

Being a university student with a learning disability put me in a situation where I could get on committees and speak to people about education issues. I had the opportunity to try to make some changes for the better in the way things are done. Many of my peers haven't had that opportunity. For me that's a little bit of reward that makes up for all of the things that I feel when I have to feel stupid.

There can also be a halo effect that comes along with being labelled learning disabled. Some people are aware of the image that advocacy organizations have pushed, that learning disabled persons are capable, creative individuals with above average intelligence. Sometimes professors automatically assume that you are amazingly talented and eager to learn. Employers may assume that you must be hardworking and resourceful in dealing with any challenge. You must be tough and have everything figured out about your disability or you would never have completed your education. There's a danger in those generalizations of course, but it's nice to have a halo once in a while.

Disclosure

There's no denying it's a difficult process, but I think I do better than most at telling people about my learning disability. I don't like to do it. It's just not that easy to say to people that you have a disability. Basically I feel that if I don't tell people, they are going to find out anyway, probably at an embarrassing moment when I'm going to be asked to write or spell something. I've tried just going along quietly, but it usually results in some situation that is incredibly awkward for everyone. To avoid those scenes and just to get it over with, I usually try to let people know right off the top. Sometimes it's the first thing out of my mouth and that's not always a good idea either, especially if you're talking to a potential employer.

In my experience, your learning disability doesn't stop being an issue just because you've disclosed your situation. People who've known me for the longest time and know all about my learning disability will still ask me to spell things or to write something down. You can't prevent those awkward moments. I've become good at making that little offhanded joke that can make everybody feel comfortable, but still makes my point. Humour helps me. If you don't laugh about some of those frustrating moments, you are going to cry. It's better just to make a joke. Then it doesn't become a big issue.

When people know about your disability, it can limit what they think you are capable of doing. Sometimes the people I know well or the people I grew up with are my worst supporters. They don't take me seriously in the way strangers will. They always question what I can and cannot do. It's bad enough that I do that. You don't want people always thinking of you in terms of what you can't do. It isn't helpful to discuss things with people who mainly see you as someone who can't read or write very well. That is the down side of disclosure. People won't hand you responsibility as readily. They're not as sure if you are capable of taking on the job at hand. Employers will tell you that the word disability worries them. They start thinking about problems right away.

The result is that I am always out there proving myself. I don't feel that there's a day that I can take off. Everywhere I go, I have to declare my situation. I can't just be like everybody else. Sometimes I know I over-compensate. Every day I feel that I've got to show why I'm there, or why I belong, or what I know. In every new situation, I have to figure out who to tell, how to tell, and how to compensate for my poor writing and spelling. I dread the arrival of forms. I find it really hard to relax, be myself, and do the best job that I can. The more anxious I am, the more dyslexic I feel. I have to convince myself and reassure myself that this situation will be okay for me. There are places where I feel accepted. Then it's really easy to be who I am. When you're in a place like that you have a chance of showing what you can do.

One of my psychology professors asked me an interesting question. "If the world would accept persons with disabilities as normal, functioning people, and they allowed them to accommodate themselves according to the way that they learn, would they be disabled?" I couldn't answer then and I still can't. The problem I see is that you do learn a set of strategies to deal with your disabilities, but they are only good in a limited set of scenarios. To live a full life you have to be able to transfer those strategies to new situations and new groups of people. It's not always an obvious process. If people didn't know what I was dealing with, it would be a distinct disadvantage for me.

My feeling is that a lot of children who are learning disabled grow up having to carry a whole lot of baggage with them before they ever get to a place where they can relax and feel accepted. I don't think labelling is the issue. Whether they are labelled or not, the reality of their difference is carried with them in their self-confidence and how they feel about themselves everywhere they go. I think what I've ended up believing is that labelling is one thing and disclosure of that label is another. Disclosure comes down to an individual's choice. I know for me, right now, disclosure is the right choice. Maybe in ten years it won't be. I think it's time and place and who you are that determines your decision.

In the world as it exists today, it has been very important for me to have the disability label. Having my situation named allowed me to learn how to deal with it more effectively. It allowed me access to services and resources that I needed. Let's face it, I had those problems whether they were labelled or not. They don't go away just because you don't name them, and sometimes avoiding labels means you are denied support and training that could make a big difference to you. Why don't we name those differences so the person can have a way of dealing with it? I wouldn't have graduated from university if I hadn't identified myself as learning disabled. It opened doors and made things possible that allowed me to succeed.

THE VIEW FROM OUTSIDE

Meeting Jay always seems to be a memorable experience. He has a big, friendly presence. There is always lots of noise and laughing around him. He stands out in a crowd and usually leaves you shaking your head and smiling. He is devoted to politics, history, sport and education. He soaks up information from television, the newspapers and all of the hot-stove experts he can find. There is hardly a topic he isn't interested in, or a person he wouldn't strike up a conversation with. He has an amazing auditory memory. He can quote parts of lectures long after the presenter has forgotten their content. You cannot fail to recognize the presence of a lively and engaged intellect. It may be sometime before you realize that Jay is severely learning disabled, but you can tell immediately that he is exceptional.

Entering university, Jay's literacy skills were at the grade three and four level. His IQ scores were impressive for the peaks and valleys, though not for the aggregate sum. His high school grades were just enough to gain him entrance, because his areas of strength were offset by his areas of weakness. He was certainly going to need more than his boundless enthusiasm to get him through his studies.

Jay came from an area with few formal resources for students with disabilities, but in his small community he had found people who recognized his abilities and helped him find ways to manage school. He had spent an extra year in high school to improve his marks and prepare himself for university work. He told me later that his huge advantage was a mother who refused to let him give up, even if it meant chasing him out the door to school. Jay had clearly internalized this determination and commitment to education, along with a positive way of looking at situations that allowed him to see possibilities rather than defeat. He was highly motivated to take on the challenges of university, but he suspected that there was no way to hide his conspicuous academic weaknesses. He was unsure of the ways to express his talents, so he quickly set out to find the people and the techniques that would help him succeed.

I was one of the people that Jay found. He was eager to talk about his learning style and study strategies. His excellent verbal skills, problem solving abilities and auditory memory made him an ideal participant in sorting out a learning plan. He loved talking about the puzzle of learning. Analyzing and improving his learning performance was exactly what he wanted to do. Jay never missed one of our weekly sessions. He gathered feedback from a variety of sources and seemed very adept at recognizing situations where he could learn well. He was an honest observer and a measured reporter of his triumphs and failures. There was always much to talk about and in this world of spoken exchange he was a very quick learner. He met adversity with patience and a sense of humour that allowed him to reassess his situation and move forward. I never doubted that Jay carried with him all of the frustrations and fears that come with being severely dyslexic, but he clearly wanted to carry them in a way that displayed optimism and strength. We laughed a great deal. We talked baseball, politics and ideas as we explored the academic and social issues that affected him. We still do.

University life gave Jay the opportunity to specialize in his strengths, both inside and outside of the classroom. He no longer had to survive math and science courses. He could join community activities that matched his interests and allowed him to maintain his confidence and make friends. But university is a print-dominated environment. The institution assumes a high level of comfort and facility in dealing with the written word. For most people print is a quick and efficient way of communicating ideas, remembering and organizing things. This was not the case for Jay. He hardly ever relied on print to support his learning or daily routines. In fact, he tried to avoid it. With print he was stuck back at struggling to decode the words in a passage, unless he already had a good idea of the content. He was very adept at using contextual clues to reason his way through the print. His writing skills were extremely limited. He didn't take lecture notes himself because it interfered with his ability to listen. Phone messages and reminder notes were hard for him to decipher, even if he found them. Dealing with print was Jay's major challenge at university, although not his only one.

It was amazing to watch Jay create an auditory learning environment for himself. He found plenty of ways to hear information. He attended lectures faithfully and rarely missed a guest speaker. He joined clubs, went to films, rented videos, and watched the news and documentaries on television. He went to workshops and haunted late night discussion groups. He used the office hours that professors offered to discuss course work and projects. His friendships always involved lengthy discussions about courses and the ways of the world.

Jay could unobtrusively increase ways of hearing information, but showing what he had learned in print to his instructors was a very big challenge. The discrepancy between the quality of the discussion Jay could have with his professors and what he could put down on paper was striking. The contrast was so great that simply by being himself he made the case for alternate ways of testing. When one of his professors offered him the opportunity to tape record his exam answers, a whole new world opened up. Jay recognized immediately the important potential that dictating his exams and papers provided. If this was a legitimate method of working at university, then he had finally found a great equalizer. He was ambitious academically and he didn't want to be relegated to the borders of failure because of his writing skills. At last there was a way for him to participate in formal education and earn grades that matched what he knew.

Free of the struggle with print Jay expressed his ideas in a richness of language and detail that was not possible otherwise. Dialogue was how he learned and demonstrated his intellectual abilities best. Interacting with a person provided an opportunity for feedback and direction during the process of creating his responses. It made learning personal and immediate. An audience didn't make him anxious. It helped him focus and produce. He excelled at finding ways of making the learning and evaluation process into a dialogue. It was an important part of his success at university. It also made him a wonderful educator for our program. Soon almost all of his teachers were firm believers in the reality of learning disabilities and the need for alternate ways of testing.

Jay worked hard at developing his skills with the dictaphone. Earning good marks by dictating your exams and papers requires more than a stream of consciousness approach. Even if you are very articulate, you can't just start talking and expect to get an A. Jay had to work on focusing and organizing his ideas to structure a high-quality argument. Some of this he learned from instruction in his

English courses and from the extra workshops he attended. The debating society and student government meetings gave him even more practice. He used feedback from the dictatypist and professors' comments on his work. Many of his writing techniques he gathered from listening to lectures. He was keenly aware of the way in which professors structured and presented their arguments. He listened to the spoken word with the sensitivity that a good reader brings to print.

Even though the dictaphone was an incredibly enabling tool for Jay, he did not stop trying new strategies. With some professors, he tried oral exams. Other times he wrote exams with his classmates and then discussed his answers with the professor following the testing session. He was willing to take the risk of trying something new, and willing to explore the suggestions offered by his professors to accommodate their teaching and evaluation preferences. Discussing learning strategies was one of the ways that he established a cooperative climate and working partnership with his professors.

The provincial rehabilitation services sent Jay a computer, but I am sure the way that he used it was not what they had expected. Problems with keyboard coordination, plus his spelling and grammar difficulties, made the computer a very cumbersome support. There was no adaptive software. Rather than letting the computer go unused, Jay dictated his ideas to a friend who typed them onto the computer. Later his friend was free to type his own papers onto the computer with Jay offering suggestions. Even though he wasn't a master of keyboarding skills Jay saw immediately how he could use the technology that he was given. This incident was typical of his ability to see beyond the immediate obstacles and find a way to participate. This problem-solving style continues to be hugely enabling for him.

At university Jay developed his strengths and was able to improvise strategies that allowed him to capitalize on his talents and minimize the impact of his disabilities. He was a genius at last minute saves, and resilient enough to withstand the stress and setbacks he encountered until a way to succeed emerged. In most situations his good natured enthusiasm made the people around him willing to pitch in and help him out. This approach certainly had an emotional cost for Jay and his supporters, but it was a price he was willing and able to pay. Effective partnerships with both professors and students were one of Jay's trademarks. He was an expert at negotiating and exchanging skills. He combined the social and the academic borrowing currency from one to assist with the other.

In spite of the relentless pace of life at the university, Jay was stubborn enough to refuse to take a reduced course load to make his life easier. He was not used to slowing down and proceeding in an orderly fashion through a reasonable work load. He was used to crisis management. To him it was safer and more forgiving. As his counsellor, it was difficult for me to watch him work himself to exhaustion rather than cut back. Jay was forced to accept that he had to do things differently than his peers, but he refused voluntarily to be slow. His goal was to earn respect for his abilities and excel. Failing to keep up was not an option. He was determined not to be separated from the group of people he admired and regarded as his peers, and he wasn't.

Was it a realistic goal for Jay to come to university? Many people didn't think so and there were many traditional indicators to support them in that conclusion (schooling experiences, high school grades, IQ scores, age at diagnosis, literacy level, socioeconomic background, and availability of resource support). You would not have predicted a successful outcome from those factors. The cluster of abilities and personal strengths that he used so effectively would have been hidden from view. Jay did much more than survive at university. His grades improved dramatically and his successes didn't stop with writing a thesis. He was a mentor and a tutor for other students and a founding participant in our transition workshops. He became an active, award-winning, honours graduate who contributed a great deal to our community.

In spite of how he may have appeared through the filter of institutional measures, Jay is one of those talented, resilient individuals who is determined to find a place and a way to excel. At university he became an effective self-advocate and an advocate for changes in educational policy for students with disabilities. For the whole of his school life, Jay has had to think seriously about the learning process and what it means to be a person with a disability. His thoughtful comments on his personal progress and his struggles make it easy to see why he was often asked to be a keynote speaker at workshops and conferences. They also made him an excellent student senator and representative in the provincial alliance of student associations. His story makes a strong case for looking beyond the deficits that define learning disabilities, to the strengths and skills that these students possess. Facilitating the development and expression of those talents and competencies can change the picture from struggle to success.

11
JAY SIMPSON
World of Work

Several times Jay and I have taped interviews about life after university. Jay is a terrific story teller. He claims that he could tell lots more stories but they would all be a variation of the same themes, so we've decided to stop and put some of them into print. Jay is an experienced teacher now. His strategies are "tried and true". He works with children struggling to learn in school. Reframing difficult situations and implementing creative solutions are a routine part of his daily life and now his career. He takes on the tough problems and the big issues. He is always on the lookout for new technology and his knack for locating funding means that there is usually an innovative project or two also on the go. He hasn't lost his gift of finding mentors and collaborators. Good working relationships with his colleagues and his students are the foundation for his success. Making education count for students keeps him going and he celebrates their success. It's his purpose. Jay is always too busy and stressed but I don't think he would have it any other way. See what you think.

Finding a Career

When it came to putting my skills to work for me in a career, I thought about being a lawyer or a social worker but it was an education program that accepted me. Some people didn't think it was a good idea for me to try for a career in teaching. Some students with learning disabilities who have tried teaching did not have the easiest time. Admissions officers will tell you the best chances for success in a training program are a passion for the work and a history of positive experiences in the area. Maybe that was me and education? Also coaching kids had been an important part of my life for fourteen years. I love working with kids. I probably am a kid but the university had hired me to work on a project mentoring and tutoring students with learning disabilities and it ended on the plus side. Then there was my experience in community education as a workshop leader and as a keynote speaker. Besides, I had shown my passion for learning in my own education. For years I had thought about learning and teaching so that I could make adjustments and be successful. Teaching sounded like it might be a good fit even if there were obvious challenges.

At the start of the education program I didn't know how I was going to deal with my learning disability as a classroom teacher. I had a good idea of my strengths and weaknesses as a learner. I had done well at university but I was the student not the teacher. I always liked that quote about knowable and unknowable unknowns. Everyone laughs at it but the truth is there are only some things that we can truly know and lots of things that you can't. For example, it's a knowable that I should not be a 911 operator or a stock boy. Those skills just aren't there and they are not going to be. I couldn't predict how I would manage in the classroom but school was a knowable unknown for me. It was a place where I had been successful and I thought I knew the system well enough to be able to change things that didn't work for me. I had been doing that for years. There were people around me who believed in me and would support me when the unpredictable problems came along. Many things are possible if you have good support.

I was an early arrival at the school of education. Most of the faculty felt that in principle there should be places for students with disabilities but implementing that kind of policy was something we all had to work on. Professors were busy teaching how to teach. They hadn't necessarily thought through how disabilities might affect a student in their own class. They didn't really expect a student with a learning disability to be there. Neither my professors nor the mentors in the classroom had ever dealt with something like this before, and neither had I. We needed a lot of discussions about what was reasonable accommodation, especially for the practicum placements. They were relatively short term. They involved a lot of different environments and demands with not a lot of time for trial and error. I was being evaluated not just on what I knew but on how I could deliver information and support learning in others. It was very different from succeeding in lecture-based courses.

I needed all of the determination and negotiating skills I possessed in order to show that I would be a good teacher. It was a struggle to get through all of the issues that came up in accommodating my learning disability. I used help from my allies and friends. The experience made me aware that some very negative attitudes toward learning disabilities were still out there. Sometimes I tried to build awareness and other times I just tried to get through. I am sure I challenged many people to think again about what it means to be a teacher. It was very stressful for me, and my health suffered, but I qualified to be a teacher.

Being a Teacher

As it turned out, teaching was a career where I had good ideas and I could manage my challenges. There are many ways to be a good teacher. My primary goal is always not to short-change my students. I strive to provide a place for learning where students can feel safe and find things that they like or are interested in. I want my students to understand who they are as learners. How do they work best? What makes them work? If they know those things, they can translate their success into their next environment. I'm prepared to use whatever tools are available to help them reach that goal. What can I do to open up those channels for learning and communication? I'm always looking to see how I might be able to do that better or differently. That's what's exciting and it keeps me going.

My focus changes but good ideas always keep coming around to me and I adapt them to the current problem. When you have a student who isn't learning, I'm the one with an idea to try. I can write a winning grant proposal so we can test out my good ideas. When you need to raise money for the school, I'm the one who knows how to make more money with less effort. I know that I have deficits. There are days when I think I should be someone else or do something else. Then I remind myself that if I were a plumber or a carpenter or something else, there would be parts of those jobs that I wouldn't like and that would be challenging for me. I try to find answers before my deficits become an issue.

Knowing is my power. I'm always observing other teachers in search of good role models to push me and compete with me in a comfortable way. That keeps me at the top of my game. I am always asking questions and looking for answers. I can't stop collecting new ideas. I got some great ideas about how to handle reluctant teachers on my team after reading how Abraham Lincoln led his team of rivals. I borrow ideas from reading and what I hear on the radio and TV. I want to know what's happening in science and religion as well as education and technology. I have this gift for storage of information. I can't necessarily tell you who told me or where I got the information but it stays there and I seem to be able to use it in the right situation. Once, my co-workers gave me a t-shirt with the motto "Research Says".

When I'm working with students, I run into my walls every day. Maybe not every day anymore, but I run into them enough that it reminds me how often the students must be running into their walls. My evaluators always say that I am very compassionate in my dealings with the students. Because of my own background, I can see some aspects of student life that other teachers can't. I also know that you have to be careful about what you read into a situation. Their experiences are not mine and I am the teacher now.

For a long time, I was worried about becoming a teacher and not having a voice to speak in support of the students and other people who I felt were disenfranchised. I have always tried to make sure that those people have a voice. I can't forget the study of people who had been unemployed and forgot what it was like to be unemployed once they got a job. Within three months of being employed again, they had less sympathy for the unemployed than most people. They believed the unemployed were just cashing in on the system. I don't want to be like that with learning disabilities. I don't forget what it was like and I think it has paid off. Now I feel I have learned both how to hold those concerns and how to cooperate in multi-disciplinary teams.

Cracking the Lineup: Getting a Teaching Job

Teaching jobs were scarce when I graduated and I knew it would be hard to break in. While I waited to find a teaching job, I worked with different advocacy groups for people with disabilities and for seniors. I have always done a lot of coaching and volunteer work and that helped too. Probably one of the best things I did was to take graduate education courses with some teachers from my community who wanted to work in administration. I commuted to the classes with some of them and we talked about the assignments together. By taking those courses, I learned a lot and it worked out that the people doing classes with me became the people hiring for the school district. They knew my background and my ideas about education. They had seen what I could do and they wanted to hire me. Those courses and the networks of friends that I had built up helped me get a job. No question about that. Still, it took me some time to convince people that I was the best person for a teaching job.

Once I got a job as a teacher, I had to look seriously at technology because I knew it could allow me to deal with print and do my work. Unlike university, I didn't have the accommodation services of a dicta-typist, note taker or reader. I had to learn to use technology to survive. Over time I got better at using the technology and the technology itself improved and became more available. The more everyone uses technology the easier it is for people with disabilities to feel comfortable using theirs. Access and prices improve too. Technology has made a huge difference for me and it has become a competitive edge for me in winning teaching positions and keeping them.

When I started out teaching, I bought the adaptive technology I needed to succeed. I remember spending what seemed then like a lot of money. I had more computers than the school did. I knew that if I taught the way everybody else did, I wasn't going to be successful. I also recognized that some of the things I needed right from the start had to be resourced in a different way than just asking the principal. By bringing the technology with me, I had that something extra to offer rather than making an extra demand.

Adaptive technology was the answer for many of my challenges but as a teacher, I wasn't just interested in technology for myself. Using technology makes ripples. You know the idea of making ripples in a pond. There are those little actions that make the whole surface different. I'm always making ripples. That's part of what I have to offer. I was interested in using technology with the students that were in my classes. I also wanted to get the students outside of my classes and the teachers that had to teach them using it too. Now many people are trying to use technology in the way that I do and I have been there from the very start. It's great! It feels good to be the developer in a founding spot.

I found a niche teaching technology and working with students who were not succeeding in a regular class room. Teaching in special education is not a traditional set of skills. You have to want to learn yourself, if you are going to be even half-decent at it. New approaches are required since the usual techniques haven't worked for the students. One of my strengths is being able to see things and do things in a different way. That can be an advantage or a disadvantage. Sometimes something different is just what is needed and people recognize that. Other times you can't crack the line-up. When I walked in the door with those skills, at the right time and in the right place, I got a job.

This wasn't the first time that I arrived at the precise time that things were changing. When I started university, I was the first student with a learning disability in my province to receive government support for a university program. I have always been lucky like that and I like being out front on the cutting edge. Being early on the scene means that you get to experiment and you're allowed to fail. In the long run it's easier. As a teacher, if you develop the program, you define your own parameters. If there are things that you don't do very well, you can put them outside of your scope. When you wait until things are tried and true, there's only one way to do it. Even if you don't fit or follow that mode, you're stuck doing it that way. That's why I always want to be an early adopter on the cutting edge.

Getting on board early is the only way you can take control of things as a teacher. With my situation and my personality, I don't want things to just happen to me. I need to control the agenda in order to succeed. I don't want to be caught behind the learning curve. In a founding spot, I can provide support and solve problems for others who will in turn support me. Leading the way is where I am comfortable and where I have the most to offer.

Talking About a Disability

Declaring my disability was one of the big things that I learned about at university. I think understanding yourself and what you can do is the first step. After that you can be comfortable explaining to someone else. In an employment situation, you also have to be able to show that you can shape the environment so that it works for you and for them.

Sometimes it seems like it would be easy to get ruled out of contention for a job if you disclose your disability. I had been warned about that even before I graduated from university. My sisters and other people I've come across have had some bad luck with declaring their disability. People did use it against them. Because of who I am as a learner, I can't really hide my disability anyway. I certainly can't hide from it in my work. How and when to disclose are the only questions open for me.

I think disclosing your disability works best when you can highlight something you can do that other people may not. Schools are excited about me because I'm trying to grasp how technology works in the real world and how this stuff is going to affect students. If I present myself in the same way as everybody else does, I believe my chances of getting a job would be very different. If I was just another resource teacher, the skills and abilities I could list would be okay but I tell them how I stand out. I show them I'm on the cutting edge and I am excited about the work I do.

It's always tough to do an interview. I've just been through the process of disclosure and selling myself again. I wanted to find a job in a different school board to be closer to my partner. I have to say it was a lot easier for me interviewing this time knowing that I had some years of experience and good references. I laid it all out on the line in the interview and I told them what I bring to the table. "As a learner and as a teacher I know myself. Over time, I have worked out what my niche is in education. If you like it and want to support me this is what I have to offer." I was able to declare that and it was true. It wasn't always like that, but now I can walk into an interview and know what I have to offer. Now I believe I can get that job if it's the right one for me.

I may be more confident but I still had to answer the usual questions all over again. How can you do the job if you have a learning disability? How can you teach reading and spelling if you can't read and spell yourself? That part doesn't go away. Usually the questions are framed in a careful way but that's what the people doing the hiring want to know. You have to be able to calmly explain. I had stories and examples ready. At the same time, you also have to be trying to figure out what kind of support you might find in the job if they do hire you.

In a job interview there are a whole lot of things you can't control. The format for the interview and the people who are on the interview team, each have a role in your success, even though those people may not be the ones that you would work with in the day to day. This last time I just happened to be interviewed by a team that included the adaptive technology person for the district. I think it made a difference. Though I didn't know it at the time, another big difference was the principal who was on the interview team. I found out later that this principal had a lot of experience with students with learning disabilities. He had done some of the first programs in his area and he had seen many of the students he worked with go on to be successful in their careers. He gets it. He saw that I had the approach they wanted. I was excited about working with him. I guess we both thought it would be a good fit. I earned myself a chance at a new school.

First Impressions

Disclosing my disability doesn't end with a successful job interview. The next challenge for me at any new school is selling myself to my co-workers. This hasn't changed. My disability is always going to appear and this last time it did almost immediately, even before classes started. Surprise! They had the whole school staff together in one room to do a grammar assessment. I was asked to sit there and do that test with everybody else. I don't do grammar and I don't feel good being put in a situation like that. If I'm not declared and I opt out, then it looks like I'm trying to avoid work and that is one thing I do not do. I felt trapped and uncomfortable. I thought, "Well, here I go already!" There were people there who knew about my situation and might well have spoken to me in advance about accommodation but they didn't. I sat there and suffered through it but I was reminded of the work I would have to do to find a place in that school.

This new job was the first time in a long while that I was about to start working with people who didn't know me. In my old school district, I had established a kind of exchange network. I had people that I could go to if I got stuck. If I needed help, they were there. I had a buddy who would edit work if I needed it. I had a cadre of people who understood and would help. I've always been lucky like that. When I moved, I lost that network. It was a big loss personally and professionally and I really felt it that day.

First impressions are important. "Every time you make a first contact, you have the ability to shape the opinions and the views that people will hold about you and your workplace from that moment on." That's a quote from the president of KLM Airlines that I picked up somewhere and it stuck with me. If every first contact is an opportunity, I decided I would take control and get started by making a presentation to the rest of the staff. I didn't want to repeat the grammar test experience. I negotiated for my chance to make the right impression at the first staff meeting.

I already knew it was a tough crowd but I got up and gave my presentation. I was nervous and over-tired from re-writing my talk multiple times, and from waiting to present it. Then it happened. I was talking about Anne, my teacher in Grade 8. I was saying how she changed my life and I started crying right in the middle of the presentation. What a way to start! Here I come into this new environment as a resource professional and I declare myself and I cry. How would I dig myself out of this one? You know I probably alienated a big bunch of people in that meeting but for those who wanted to hear what I had to offer, it was probably the most authentic thing I could have done.

To finish off my day, the vice-principal tells me that his wife has a learning disability and that she is a very successful principal. He wanted me to know there would be no excuses. He said he was a hard-driving personality and he was going to call me out if I wasn't organized enough. I thought, "Oh my, we are in for a bad year!"

Keeping the Job

When I started my new job, I was basically swimming under water. For years I had been in a system where, over time, I had been able to create an environment that worked for me. I wasn't sure I could do it again. I told myself this was my chance to be a new teacher again. Here was the opportunity to reset and re-examine my practice. I hoped I could rely on technology and some of my usual strategies to get me through.

Right away I found a piece of software that I thought would help the students with learning disabilities. It allowed multiple student users and supported them with spelling when I couldn't. I called England and I spent my own money to have them send it over. That was a start. I was also supposed to teach phonics. The research says that working on synthetic phonics really helps kids with learning disabilities. I have trouble hearing the sounds you need to teach phonics. If I can't hear them, I can't teach them. I found the program that could but I was already working on writing another technology grant. I couldn't apply for two, so I found a teacher who I thought might be able to use the program as well. After we talked about it, she was willing to apply for the phonics grant.

Another colleague had given me all of her information about an intervention program she thought would be promising. She wanted me to try it and see if it was effective. I took that information and I wrote a proposal mixing together the use of the adaptive software I wanted with the intervention program she wanted. We got a big grant from an outside source. Now we have both the software and the intervention program. I think it was mostly because I was going to teach kids with learning disabilities. That's how I like my accommodations to work. They make things better and not just for me.

At my old school I coached basketball for a lot of years and I started coaching soccer at my new school. I'm not a great basketball or soccer coach and it takes a lot of extra time, but it doesn't matter. What does matter is that it shows the school that I am putting in an effort. It matters that your employer figures you are trying your very best. That way when you do make mistakes, and you will, they seem to be earnest and honest mistakes rather than neglectful and lazy ones. I like thinking about that play *The Importance of Being Ernest* where it really pays off to be earnest even just by name.

At first when I sat there and looked at my situation, I thought "This school isn't for me." This is not where I'm going to perform the best unless I find some collaborators. So I went searching to find people who wanted to work with me and change what they were doing. Luckily, I found some. By the time my vice-principal said he wasn't entirely impressed with my first couple of months in the school, the principal said, "Just give him some time, he'll get there."

Like the vice-principal, I hadn't been entirely impressed with the way things were going. I had to work really hard to establish myself. My partner was a teacher in the same school and she works really hard too. We were at school early every day. I was in that school every Saturday and Sunday pretty much for the first few months, but I think most new teachers are. It certainly helped. Every day, I made contacts and I said the positives. I pointed out the good things that people were doing. I tried to build relationships and I tried to get what I needed to get done in a very economical way. I kept doing little things like helping out the registrar. Then she turns out to be one of the persons deciding on hiring. I worked with all of the educational assistants and taught them how to use our technology with the students. I wanted them to know. Now everyone has profited from their learning. The principal found out about that project and he assigned twenty-five percent of my time for working on training inside the school. This meant I didn't have to travel around from school to school. That was a big bonus for me. The little things paid off.

At the end of the year, after some convincing, I agreed to be the guest speaker for a professional development session. Yes, the crying didn't stop me. By then most everyone wanted more people to hear what I had to say. I talked about disclosure and the importance of self-advocacy and adaptive technology. There were two people at that talk that really clicked with me. I didn't know at the time but one of them turned out to be the person who had more to say than anyone about who gets hired and how the teaching blocks are assigned. She knew a lot about learning disabilities and she wound up being one of the people who advocated for me staying in my job. The other person turned out to be one of my best collaborators. She was chosen to be the next vice-principal at the school and wanted to work with me.

I know that I am a teacher-leader not an administrator. All of the skills you need are just not there for me to be an administrator. I also know that I need to have somebody inside the system to work with me because I can't change the things I need to change on my own. The new vice-principal was what I needed. She is an amazing person. She has a very good sense of organization and planning. That is not who I am. Our skills complement one another and we work well together. We both want to make things better for kids. When the opportunity to work with the new vice-principal for another year came along, I could see that it would be almost like going back to my old school where I first started teaching. I could use all of the lessons I learned from the experience I got back then. Maybe together we could move things forward and make some good things happen.

Two months in, if someone had told me that I'd be willing to go back to this new school I wouldn't have believed them. By the end of the year that didn't seem like such a bad idea. The school and the school board were doing whatever they could to keep me in the area. They realized the value of the set of skills that I have to offer. The big plus was that it would allow me to stay with my partner and start the process of becoming a permanent employee. I was willing to take the slings and arrows again, so I agreed to stay and take the job. I already knew that making change happen takes time and a lot of effort, but it's what I do. Now I am living and working in the same place as my partner. I guess you could say the try out was a success.

Moving Things Forward

We all know that the kids who don't fit require far more effort than the kids who fit. Keeping kids with mental health issues or keeping kids with learning disabilities means there is chaos because they've got piles and piles of baggage that they're just trying to unlock. When I work with kids with learning disabilities in my class, nine times out of ten, the learning disability is the easiest problem to deal with. What's really hard to deal with is the baggage that goes along with it. Maybe we can learn how to change the way we deal with students who don't fit and we will lose fewer kids. Once you get wrapped up in this kind of challenge, you have to see it through to the end. That can motivate you and the people you work with. It's like my days with the baseball team. Once I took over coaching, I had to see the team through to the championship in spite of all the years it took.

Systems work or don't work because people keep reproducing the same things over and over again. In all of the years I've spent in school as a student and now as a teacher, I've had to change things in the system that don't work for me. I don't think in a linear way and I am able to connect diverse ideas that other people might overlook. It means that I have lots of ideas and programs just waiting to be tried and plenty of experience at figuring out how to change a learning environment. Some of the teachers I have worked with weren't the best at finding new methods to use with their students but that doesn't mean they don't have a real passion for working with the kids.

Working together we can make good things happen. When there are people who have things to give, I can help make it count for the students. That's my purpose.

In student services, I have to be able to motivate teachers and teaching assistants to take up the challenge and find ways their students can be successful. I need them to implement individualized programs and then try again if they are not working. Some of the teachers can't and some of the teachers won't. If it's that they won't, then you have one problem and there's nothing much more you can do for them or with them. But if they can't or they are just not there yet, well then, there's a whole bunch of other things that I can do to help move them forward.

I don't have to move a whole country forward, but some days I feel like I know something of how Abraham Lincoln felt when he had to move a whole nation forward. He had a vision of how things could change and he made it happen. I was really inspired by the way he managed people, especially the ones who didn't agree with him. He understood the art of picking the right time to do things. He got people ready to hear his message. Then, he told them stories to make his points and encourage them. Those are things I try to do in my practice.

In one of my previous schools I was trying to get my colleagues to look at the principles of differentiation in the classroom. I kept talking about differentiation any chance I got. Finally, my principal told me to stop. He said people were not ready to hear about it. I stopped. Instead I got people started on a program called Young Active Readers that had material for students to work at different levels. The teachers tried it and became comfortable using it. Many of them weren't ready to take the step toward implementing a big concept like differentiation when I first raised the idea in the way I did. When I suggested using the Young Active Readers program, it had real appeal. This was the way I learned that if people have the materials and the support they need, they will be more willing and able to adopt something new. First you need a set of tools and systems to make it easy and that starts the shift to the path you want them to follow. I guess you could say that gets them ready to change. I have learned the hard way how important timing and the language you use is in making my ideas a success.

One of the teachers I work with is very good but sometimes he gets locked into a way of doing things with a student that just isn't working. I saw that he was getting frustrated so I broke off my day and I went to see him. I pointed out all of the wonderful things he has done for this particular kid. I got him to think about where he had started and where we were right now. Then he said, "I know, but I want more." I tried to convince him that sometimes you have to be thankful for what you've got. Otherwise what you're going to do is turn that student off.

When I came in after a few days with a suggestion for a new plan, it wasn't hard to sell. I told him I thought doing "app" reviews on the I-pod was something this kid was probably willing to write about. I pointed out the virtues, "It's new and interesting and it's real. It follows all the rules for success." He said "I think that might have some potential." All I did was remind him of what was there and tell him why this new plan might work for his student but I waited until he was ready to hear it. By having this conversation, I helped the student, I helped the teacher and I helped myself. All it took was investing a little time to show the successes. When we're standing right in front of things, we don't always see the whole situation. That conversation was enough to get the teacher going again. Sometimes we just need that. I've opened the door to ways for him to work for me and for my student. Nobody loses in that.

One of my teaching mentors gave me some advice that I still try to practice. Her point was that you have to come to terms with the things you can change and the ones that you can't. The schools where I have worked have taught me that not everyone wants to make a change. A person can hold on for dear life and hope to outlast whatever comes next or you can embrace the change and move with it to see where it might take you. Whatever you decide it still takes time and effort but the reality is that no matter how much you want things to stay the same, they are always going to change.

When I started teaching, not everybody wanted the changes that I wanted to make but with a group of supporters we learned how to make it happen. We made the school a better learning environment for more kids. I want to be able to move things forward like that no matter where I work. Whatever little bit I've been able to accomplish in making this change, the credit goes to those people I have worked with. I know there is a phrase, "We stand on the shoulders of giants." I don't think you need a giant to stand on. You just need a system that allows people to give the best of what they have to offer. Well, maybe with a little push too.

Working Relationships

How do I get people to work with me? Ever since I began teaching, I seem to be able to find amazing people who are really good at what they do and we start working together. Those partnerships are a big part of my success. With those people I was allowed to ask, "What do you do well?" I recognize their strengths. Then they do the things that they do well and I get to do the things that I do well. It works out so that together we meet the needs of the students. I've learned to accommodate myself by accommodating other people. I seem to manage to find or create an environment that allows that to happen.

At university I learned a lot about negotiating for accommodations. I could use the hammer of policy and legal rights to get what I needed, like a lot of my friends did. Or I could use the reasonable choice method and convince people to make a fair accommodation. If you negotiate the right way, then you can always come back and ask again. If you do it the wrong way and create bad feelings, you can only ask once or as long as the hammer is in your court. The next time the hammer is in their court, I guarantee they will be using the hammer on you.

Sometimes I spot people to work with me or my ideas draw them in. One of my principals told me that I was like a lightning rod. I have the capacity to load energy into other people in a way that gets them charged and ready to engage. In the beginning it wasn't always that way but I'm passionate about what I do. When you are like that, other people get involved too. If there is artistry to what I do, it's painting pictures with other people. I don't paint alone.

One of the big stressors for me is paperwork. No matter what job I have or course I take I always have to worry about the paper work involved. I know it will eventually get done. I will find a way through. Unfortunately, it seems the province that hires me as a teacher has a very different view on that. They are serious about their deadlines and they don't see me as qualifying for secretarial support. I know I have technology to help me but I often need a person to be the secretary for meetings or edit and put the finishing touches on my reports. Until I find the partners I need, my stress levels go off the charts.

With my diagnosis I don't necessarily read people very well. But there is one thing that I get implicitly and I teach it to the students with autism. I talk about the bank. You put things into the bank and you take things out of the bank. If you don't put anything into the bank there isn't anything to take out. I always make sure to put something in. I have created this systematic approach in my work environment. I do the same things all the time. I always make sure that I'm trying to be accommodating and trying to be generous of spirit. That's not hard for me. I think I'm that way anyway.

In my classroom space, I try to partner with the people around me but I don't take advantage of them. I get them to help me but I also help them. It might mean that someday I'll stay until 4:30 to help you learn this really great computer program. Or I might let your kid use my I-Pad while we are having a meeting. I have a decent set of skills around technology that I can offer. Sometimes it's something else. With one teacher I explain how to work transitioning into her classroom. For another teacher who doesn't like talking on the phone to parents, I can do that for her. What I do is mutually beneficial.

Sometimes I feel like a blunt instrument, but when I work with others, I am able to motivate them so good things get done. I can't always be the person to sit there and make things happen but I've always been able to work well with the teaching assistants. They are the most important tools that I have. I identify what they are good at and I tell them that they are good at it. I'm the first person to say "I think you've done a good job." I'm empathetic. I appreciate their situation. Sometimes I think they have the worst job in the whole school. I wouldn't want to be in a job where my ideas weren't heard. I want to listen to them and I want to give them a voice. I tell them what they are doing is important.

When you do that, and you thank them, all kinds of good things happen. You'd be surprised at how many people don't do any of those things. When people feel like they are being appreciated and listened to, they see things that they didn't see before. I come in and say, "I really like this about what you're doing, and I'm wondering what it is that you want to do next?" Then we talk. They buy in and do great work with the students. Some people don't think we need to support professionals that way, but I need to move people and I believe the best way to do that is to let them see their own way forward. In my field it is important to care and be passionate about the work not just with the students.

Once I am able to get a group of assistants working together for the students, they support me and help me. My classroom gets decorated and cleaned up. They do all kinds of things that probably keep me in a job. I guess the skill has been to find the personal wins for myself by recognizing the value of other people. Five of the assistants I've worked with have become teachers. I'm very proud of them and their success. Sometimes I think what I've shown them is that anybody can do it.

With my teaching colleagues I can't be rigid and I can't be a stick in the mud. I cultivate a personality of being flexible. They all know that I will be willing to do what has to be done to make things work. The idea is that others will then be flexible with me when I need it. This exchange is not hard for me. I want to be a nice guy. I like doing these things anyway. I'm not just looking to line up favours. I know sometimes people take advantage but I rarely mind as long as I am the one who has chosen to do more than my share.

Teachers sometimes have problems with some of the people they work with. I will see these same issues but I don't let it affect the way I work. I just continue and move on with what I am doing. If I'm slighted or annoyed, I have to get over it quickly. There are just as many people that I don't like but I look for that part of them that I can like. I can't hold on to those other things because I have to work with them. I've got to look for the offsets. I don't get a choice. My world view is different and I need good relationships to succeed. Once you determine that you don't get a choice, it's easier to accept the reality in front of you and just carry on.

This idea of being different but really the same is a hard one to deal with. Yes, I'm different but I'm also the same because everybody carries issues and problems. Because I'm a resource teacher, I'm not one with the classroom teachers. Because I have a learning disability, I'm not one with teachers either. My math is weak and my spelling is awful and so on. I don't feel I belong. I always feel like I'm at odds with my identity. In some ways that is useful. As a resource teacher I have to work with every teacher in the school and potentially any student in the school. I need people to work with me and for the students. I try not to take sides and I try to be as fair as possible. If I'm perceived to be with one group or another group then it really affects how people will deal with me. I avoid conflict and that means I don't have to always be in that fight or flight situation with other people. I try to create good will instead. That way I can be honest and say things that other people might not be able to. My suggestions can't be underestimated or dismissed as playing politics. I'm the honest broker.

Way back in my undergraduate years, I heard the statistic quoted that fifty per cent of graduate students felt counterfeit and like they didn't really belong. I was thinking about that the other day when I was listening to a radio program on identity. They interviewed the guy from Anonymous who is the only one in Anonymous that everybody knows. Then there was the man who wrote about being First Nations and being white and not really belonging to either group. They pointed out that for all of us there is always that feeling of being 'in' and 'out' at the same time. That's the way I am in my job as a teacher and the way I am as a person. I'm 'in' and 'out' in all groups. What I'm trying to do now is remove that layer that keeps me feeling like an outsider.

Personal Life

If you think my relationship skills work pretty well in the work environment, you are right. They do but when it came to dating it was a different story. The rules at work are relatively simple. When I work with my kids with autism, I understand what's happening but dating is complicated. I don't necessarily read people well if I haven't spent a lot of time with them. Dating is about reading and reacting to people you don't know very well. By the time that I've spent enough time with someone to get to know them I've probably developed another kind of relationship with them.

When it came to dating it seemed much harder to figure out when or how to continue. It's like a drug shoots through you and prevents you from looking for all the things you know you're supposed to be looking for. It takes a lot of practice and in the world of dating you don't want to be hurt or to hurt anyone else. I'm not afraid to try and I'm not afraid to fail in the work situation, but on a personal level it's different. Most of the people that you are meeting are in your environment so the risk is that you destroy a relationship or create something awkward that you have to live with. Maybe that's why most people practice when they are teenagers.

I spent a lot of time avoiding dating. I felt it was better to put work ahead of my personal life. It just made more sense to me but as time passed, I realized that I had to start taking some risks. I didn't want to spend the rest of my life without a family of my own. My friends talked me into trying computer dating. One more time technology helped me out. It was a good way to start. Encountering people in a dating situation was a new experience. I learned a lot and I met people I really enjoyed. I realized dating wasn't that scary.

I have a partner now. This is a big change for me. When we wanted to move in together and have a family, we were both teaching but we were in school districts miles apart. The distances meant that commuting wasn't an option. When I agreed to try teaching in my partner's area, it felt like a very big risk. I would be starting all over again but I knew that things wouldn't work out for us if I couldn't be happy at work. Teaching is what I do and how I identify myself. It is just such a big part of my life and my identity that it would have to be the determining factor. I have planned my life around my career right down to taking courses every year all through my summer vacation.

Knowing that about myself means my career has to affect the decisions that I make. If I could be happy and successful working in a new job I would stay.

Against the odds, I got a job in my partner's school district and I was able to negotiate a leave from my permanent role. It was hard to start over. Friends and relationships have always been a big part of my life and my success. I miss the old friends that I have known forever and who know me all too well. I got locked out of the house the other day. I forgot the keys. I had no one to call. I'm not used to that. I have made lots of work friends but I've only made one friend outside of work. I'm still no good at household things. I find it hard to keep track of the details and to find the energy to do chores after a day at work. When we went looking to buy a house in the trendy new suburb my partner spotted, I despaired of ever finding my way home. All of the houses looked the same to me. We bought one and painted it red and I haven't been lost once. I'm not that easy to live with but I've found out that I have a partner who mostly doesn't mind.

Moving has given me a new understanding of the resources I have in my personal life and as a teacher. At work I was surprised at how receptive people were to me and my ideas. I was afraid that my skills wouldn't be recognized or valued. It has been empowering to use my strengths in a new situation. I wasn't sure I could fit into a new environment but I have managed even in some very challenging situations. I expected more of a struggle to prove myself but I've been able to reproduce my success as a teacher and have a personal life as well. It has turned out that moving schools has been good idea.

Resilience

What if you're not in the right place? Maybe you want to move schools. Maybe you get reassigned or get a new supervisor. Things change, especially in a school district. There are times when you have to force yourself into a place that doesn't meet your needs. It's a hard road to shape or fit into that kind of environment. Those times are not going to be the highlights of your career because you are in an uphill battle and you already have a struggle with your disability. We've all seen what happens when you fight on two fronts and no one gives you any grace or gratitude. You're very limited. Your life is very different when you find a place where you fit and your skills are valued and needed.

Sometimes the context for my teaching changes in ways that don't seem like a good fit for me. I think of myself as a teacher-leader but in some of those situations, I found it very difficult to imagine how I would manage to provide resource support let alone lead. I didn't always know if I could establish new partnerships in the positions I was given. From baseball, I knew that if you lead a team well, you do the little extra things that open the door for people to find the right place to contribute to the team and get some wins. I always try to do that and so far, the strategy has worked pretty well. I have been able to negotiate my way through the differences, but that doesn't mean that I didn't have a lot of angst about some of those changes.

I am a teacher and I have found my niche as a resource and technology specialist but what if they assign me to a classroom? One of my friends, a principal I used to work for, doesn't think I should worry. He always tells me, "Where you're planted, you will bloom." I am not entirely convinced. Maybe I can fit in a classroom, but it's got to be the right classroom. This year I taught a little bit in the classroom. The class in art (not my area) went surprisingly well and baseball was a gift. The relationships that I created with the students made things work out. This year and with these courses it worked, but I wouldn't want to push things much further. I think if I were to teach in a classroom on a regular basis my biggest allies would be my students. Even then, it would have to be the right kind of classroom.

To manage a classroom in the long term, I would need to be in a bigger high school where I could teach the same course multiple times. In the little school districts where you teach seven different classes or an elementary classroom where you have more than twenty students and multiple subjects to teach them, it wouldn't work for me. What it basically boils down to is that those classrooms require so much preparation and so much organizational time that it would be too overwhelming for me. I think that's part of knowing yourself and not ignoring the reality of your disability.

Here's another example. What do I do when my school decides to focus on mathematics teaching as their program development priority? That is not me. You would know how true that is if you saw my psycho-educational assessment. I knew there was no way I could figure out myself how to improve our programming in this area. I decided to try wrangling a bunch of people to answer that question. My hope was that people with better math minds than me would get excited about participating in the new plan and something very good would happen. I found people who had the ability to start gathering good resources. I could lead the way by asking good questions. My other contribution was offering ways we could use technology and the internet as part of the process. I know it's a cliché, but by working together, we came up with some exciting new ideas.

The worst thing you can do is lie to yourself and try to be what you are not. You are what you are and if that is not good enough, you're probably not in the right spot. That's easier to say now that I have some experience and I am in a spot where I have contractual rights to compete for a collaborative environment and a place that wants what I have to offer. There are days that I don't do as well as I want to. There are days that are awful. You fail like everybody else does but you keep on trying. Growing up with the idea that everyone thought I was being lazy, I seemed to figure out that you out work your problems. I see things in a different way. I am not a linear thinker so I am able to connect diverse ideas that other people might overlook. That means I have lots of new ideas and plenty of experience at figuring out how to change a learning environment to make it work better for everyone. That belief allows me to get by the things that I have trouble with. When I am in one of those times when I think "This will never work. I should go do something else." I can endure. We all just have to find a way to kind of push through and hope that over time your strategies and good work will pull you through. That's the resilience piece.

I remember reading the John Irving book, *Prayer for Owen Meany*. It was about learning disabilities in a whole bunch of different ways. The narrator was a man who was learning disabled and he was writing about a boy who was learning disabled and the author is learning disabled too. The character Owen knows that there's a purpose for him and that there's a reason why he's there doing the things that he's doing. That's my myth too. Even though I might feel at odds with who I am, like the fictional Owen Meany, I have my myth and I know that there's a purpose for me.

When things don't look like they are going to go the way you want and they look like they are never going to be the way that would let you be happy, that's when you need your myth. Even if the reason is only for you, it allows you to endure. The reason I endured all the problems I had at university was the thought that I had to help every other kid with a learning disability get funding to come too. I couldn't let them down. I still can't let the others with learning disabilities down. This is my myth. I know it's a myth but it's a myth I live with because it makes me able to carry on. It is part of my resilience. You have to have a myth or something that tells you why you are here.

Looking back

Life was very different for me without access to the kind of technology that is available today. Over the years, access to technology has created a much better environment in classrooms for me and for students. When I started out as a teacher, we used my technology in the classroom. I had more devices than the school did. The standard classroom didn't even dream about having an LCD, document cameras or word processors. I remember the technology I was given at university by the provincial support services. It was a state-of-the-art, giant, desktop computer. They wanted to have it chained to a desk in the library for what they called security reasons. In the end, I 'stole' it from the library and used a friend's car to take it to my residence room so I could use it. I wasn't very good at typing so I loaned the computer to other students in exchange for their typing services. This was a long time before the spread of lap tops and personal devices so time on a computer was a worthwhile commodity to exchange. Now schools and students have all kinds of technology available to them that were certainly not there when I started out as a technology user in 1988. That's a long time ago now and technology has made a world of difference for everyone.

Even though technology is light years ahead of where it was when I left university, some other parts of being a learner don't change. I still take every professional development course on offer and technology is now my specialty but when I started another master's program, it gave me a reminder of the perspective of a student with a learning disability. It was almost like starting the whole school thing all over again. It seems it's always challenging to be in a class especially on the first day. In my essay to introduce myself and my learning goals to the professor, I wrote "I feel stupid again." Even though I can look like I really know a lot, some days I feel like I don't know anything. Being in a classroom with the prospect of being evaluated still brings out those negative feelings.

After class, the professor asked what I needed for accommodations. She said she felt really badly for me. Her son has a learning disability and she said she knew about the struggle a classroom could be. I told her that even though I am bright, I don't process information like everyone else. When the pace goes too fast, I may not be able to process very well but my partner is in the class so I can get notes and have discussions with her after class. I ask lots of questions and she can count on me for discussion. It should be fine. I don't think that conversation could have happened in the same way twenty years ago for many reasons. That's how I know things have changed.

I went into this second master's program with the goal of learning more about adaptive technology. I was also hoping to find twenty disciples who would help spread the word about using adaptive technology. Every time I talked in class, I talked about adaptive technology. Every time I present anywhere, I talk about adaptive technology. Hopefully I don't do it until everyone is nauseated but I want to share that information and get feedback from potential users. I want to be able to make the case and increase the use of technology. When every final student presentation in our class had adaptive technology in it, I felt that maybe I had made an impact. I also got my second master's degree.

This year I'm giving a presentation on adaptive technology at the provincial teacher's conference. It's the first time that group has invited me and I am hoping to find some more supporters for technology there. It seems a long way from 1988. I have been given an offer to go to China on an exchange for the summer term. To make the right fit for me, I'm actually going to have to find and fund portable technology to use in their classrooms. I'm told that's one thing they don't have in the school I would be going to. If I go, I'm going to have to bring whatever it is I need with me. I understand who I am, and I'm prepared to spend what I need to in order to make it possible to take up the opportunity. That part hasn't changed.

In my career as a teacher, I think there were places where the students didn't get the best instruction, but it wasn't because I was learning disabled. It was because I was a beginner. When you're a novice in anything, research tells us that our lack of experience means there are things we will look back on and say, "Oh my god, I can't believe I did that." Knowing what I know now, there are a lot of things that I definitely could have done better. But the only way you recognize that is if you have learned more than when you started out. I'm hoping, that if I do things right, in twenty years I'll be looking back and saying, "Knowing what I know now, I would have made some different decisions."

Looking Forward

They have asked me to stay in my current school district. I told them I would give it three years. After that I think I might want to do something else. I've always wondered about being a technology consultant. For now, it's just about managing my health. There's a cost to staying until six every night. I'm not eating the way you're supposed to and I'm not exercising. I could get away with that in my thirties but it can't happen anymore. I can't live like that either. School can't be my whole life anymore. With summer workshops, I didn't have a vacation even though I wanted a holiday and probably needed one too. School was my life and now with my partner I'm just trying to find a way to create a healthier balance for both of us.

I have been able to recreate my teaching success in a new environment and have a personal life. I wasn't sure it would be possible. My skills are much more mobile than I imagined. It's a relief to know they are. I think with switching schools in the last three years, I know myself better as a person and as a teacher. I am more aware of my assets. This new teaching position was in a good school in the heart of the geographical area where everyone wants to be. I never thought this was a job that I was going to get. There are hundreds of teachers looking and for me to get into the school seemed almost impossible. Then for the school board to want to keep me, when they have lots of resource teachers they can compare me with, seemed amazing.

I think the question for me now is "How much of yourself do you want to invest again?" It's a huge investment any time you want to make changes. I have to pick my spots and my times. I remember my friend who championed cooperative learning approaches and I saw the personal losses she experienced. In my case, I don't go to the staff room to eat. I'm in my classroom all the time. I come to work early and I go home late. It really boils down to liking what I do. A big part of that is finding people who are interested in the change that I'm trying to make and working with them to provide more success for everyone. There are sacrifices but if what you're doing is greater than you and you believe in it, then it's worth it.

Success and Failure

Some of the people I've gone to school with have done very well financially. They have risen to the top in the careers they have chosen. But I think the important questions to ask are: Where do you want to put your markers down? What is it that you want to have in your life? What kind of success do you want to have with your career? We all think about the big things, but life is really about the small things and the things that you want to have in the day to day.

I'm really interested in what I do. I'm not expert at anything but I'm not afraid to try and I'm not afraid to fail. When I say I'm not afraid to fail, I don't mean that I'm looking to fail but I'm not so concerned about things not working out that I won't try something new or different. Part of getting to know yourself better is being confronted with what you can't do as well as what you can do. At some point you figure out that different is okay, even though my differences can mean that failure is just around the corner. The reality is failure is going to happen. That's true for everyone. There's no guarantee but if you feather your nest with people who you didn't scorn when they failed, then it's more likely they won't scorn you because you failed. The people I really try not to fail are the students. I try every day to do the things that they need.

As you get older, the falsehoods that you believe about yourself start to disappear. Maybe you can accept more. You have to be careful because the accepting means that sometimes you don't run the four-minute mile, even if you could. At the same time, you can look at yourself in a realistic way and for me that means saying I'm not an administrator of a program and I don't need to be to make changes in the school. I won't get the same recognition, but I didn't get into this business to get recognition, I wanted to make change. I'm not here to make people say, "He's an awesome teacher. This is a wonderful program." I wouldn't care except for the fact that my reputation matters in the sense of getting me my pick of jobs. The better I am at my job, the more options I have to make change. The poorer I am at my job, the fewer options I have. It is all part of trying to find that place where I can be happy with myself.

I always get comments on how enthusiastic I am about what I do. I am enthusiastic because what I do excites me. It's changing things. It's my purpose. This is what I'm here to do. I always know, even when I'm down, that I'm lucky. My family's there, my partner, some old friends too. We get on the phone and it gets better. You share gallows humor and you move on. I've always had good people around me. When you are with good people and you take advantage of the things they offer, it makes success for everyone.

I have realized that part of my success is the fact that when I declare my disability, I create opportunity in my field. Maybe if you were a 911 operator it doesn't create opportunities for you, but for me it certainly has. The fact that I have been able to start making changes here in a really quick amount of time was exciting. I was able to draw on my previous experiences and it worked pretty well. Now I am on committees and I have opportunities to take on projects that I didn't imagine would be available to me, especially in a big school district.

It's nice to be the developer in a founding spot. It's good to feel you are on the cutting edge.

This year I got to go to Florida to two international technology conferences. One was looking at assistive technology for persons with disabilities and the other one was for technology in general. I realized that the things I've been doing with three other people in our region stand up very well with what is going on in best practice. The only thing that's different between us and some of the other programs is that they are openly and financially supported by the people in their school boards. We just do the best we can by improvising with what we have. We've been working hard and our school board has supported us in the sense that they didn't stop us. They just didn't have the financial wherewithal to make where we wanted to go a reality. Our support also comes from teachers working together. People that I worked with took the ideas that I had to offer and we worked together to create a model for our school.

The things that are happening here are really exciting. We've taken the resources and the knowledge we had and started to do programming, instead of just putting up our hands and saying we can't do anything. We found outside funding. We pushed the limits of the funding and what the supports allowed us to do. When you are in early days with a model you have to do what you can with what you've got. We're certainly not where we want to be but our successes stand out from our neighbours and we hope they will adopt some of our ideas. We are celebrating the little victories and that helps everyone. We'll see where things go.

When I think about whatever skills and resources I have or don't have, it reminds me of my great friend and baseball coach. He told me that when you're coaching baseball you don't have control of everything. You don't control the sky. You don't have control over what other teams you are playing. Some years you may be able to get in forty practices and other years only twenty. But when we were coaching together, whatever resources we had, we used. Sometimes it meant finding a grant to buy equipment or spending our own money to buy uniforms for the team. He told me his secret. "You leave it all on the field because that means that whatever you do you can walk away with satisfaction. Whatever tools you have on the day, if you used them all that's success." When I became a teacher, I did that and it has really worked for me.

THE VIEW FROM OUTSIDE

After you read Jay's account of his university years, what did you expect to find in the next chapter? Did you see someone who barely survived the education system of his youth and would have no legitimate place as a teacher-leader? Jay will tell you there are people who believed just that and there are still. Maybe you saw a talented and determined person who would not be shut out or relegated to the sidelines of employment. Perhaps you even expected the innovative educator who opens the doors to success for people with disabilities that Jay has become.

I was one of the people who was not convinced that teaching would be a good career choice for Jay. I never doubted that he had much to offer a traditional educational system. Many times, I had seen him educate hearts and minds about disability issues but to me, being a teacher just didn't seem like a good fit for his working life. Clearly, this shows the limits of my imagination and my optimism. I felt he would be defeated by the structures of the system and the demanding tasks of organizing and managing time. I was distracted by his deficits and underestimated the power of Jay's creative problem-solving abilities. I am delighted to see how wrong I was! Thinking of Jay's successes and struggles always makes me realize how important it is to join people with learning disabilities in their optimism and their desire to make choices that follow their interests and strengths.

It's easy to underestimate Jay when you see the obstacles he faces in the day to day. If you focus on his disabilities, you might not hire Jay to be a teacher. Yet if you listen to him, watch him with people and see him in action you realize you couldn't find a better person to teach your child and contribute to your school. I knew any school would be lucky to have him but I wasn't convinced a school would realize it or help him manage the considerable demands of being a teacher. Now we have just found out how it can happen.

Jay grew up with a passion for politics and history. He has always enjoyed debating the current issues that have the media buzzing. Teaching was not a lifelong goal for him, but in many ways, he was a natural teacher. From the moment he walked onto the university campus, anyone could see that he loved to learn and that he loved to share what he had learned. For the whole of his school life, he had to think seriously about the learning process and its many forms. At university, Jay became a successful student and wrote a thesis on the politics of funding universities. He became an effective advocate for changes in educational policy for students with disabilities. He developed his abilities as a community educator in his role as student senator, as a representative in the provincial student association and as a keynote speaker at conferences and workshops. If you consider this list of impressive achievements, rather than focussing on his deficits, why was his success as a teacher ever in doubt?

Early in his own education, Jay had found ways of adapting to inhospitable environments. Now he has learned to transform them. Adaptive technology has been a powerful tool in unlocking possibilities for him. It has given him a new level of access to information, independence and expertise. It is an important addition to his array of accommodation strategies and he has gone on to use it brilliantly to create a career specialty. At first, Jay's lack of basic literacy skills made it difficult for him to qualify for a teaching position but he has turned his learning disability into a competitive advantage. His difference works for him. He has managed to associate his difference with innovation, progress and creativity. He will tell you he didn't have a choice. "I see things in a different way. This is what I have to offer. Then it's my flexibility and determination that make my plans work out." In his schools and in his province, he is a leader working to improve the learning environment for students and teachers.

It's exciting to see how Jay has been able to transform his various workplaces and build working partnerships just as he did at university. Every day he puts his considerable skills and insights into action for his students. Jay is well aware of both his strengths and weaknesses. There is a sense of acceptance of his disability that drives him rather than limits him. When he finds himself in a new situation he is not blinded by the barriers. He looks for opportunities and resources and finds ways to orchestrate the changes he needs while setting the stage to make the learning environment better for everyone. Win/win situations are a specialty. He finds mentors and collaborators and never forgets to contribute his share in working partnerships. He is a terrific role model for his students.

As a teacher and leader of a resource program, Jay has found his career in education both a rewarding and a stressful place to be. He has paid a price for the way he "out works" his challenges. It has brought him some health issues, but school is an environment where he can thrive. His disability has taught him that nothing comes easily. He has the patience, strength and confidence to wait until even the determined doubters come around to seeing what he has to offer. It seems his basic optimism and generous spirit allows him to carry on and not lose sight of his goals.

Now Jay has a home and a family of his own in addition to his career. Even though it might seem to an outsider that Jay has been faced with a host of challenges, he sees himself as lucky and surrounded by supportive friends. He communicates his energy and enthusiasm for life and all that it involves. He works tirelessly for the happy endings that he hopes for and believes in. With few hesitations, he cheerfully accepts the role he has created as a pioneer on the cutting edge.

12
The View from the Sidelines

When I first met our contributors, they had already found ways to be successful students. Against the odds, they had managed to earn admission to university. They brought a variety of experiences and a mixed history of support and success in school. At university they refined a new set of learning and life skills and established a history of success as independent adults. We had all learned things about managing the challenges of university, but what would happen in the years that followed? Graduation meant that the supports provided by an educational institution would disappear. Would they be able to establish a career and a home base of their own? I believed in their abilities but it seemed to be a very big step with many new and diverse demands. In setting out to begin this second set of working life conversations, I was not sure what I would find. Like the parents and teachers that saw these students off to university, I wondered how they would find ways to continue their success.

It has been a very rewarding experience working with these young people first when they were enthusiastic, aspiring students and then revisiting them some twenty years later. I am delighted by the successes I see, but also reminded of the obstacles they face. Their learning disabilities have not shut them out of the opportunities that education and employment offer. They were able to build on their strengths and establish careers that matched their interests. The ability to deal with the adversity in their lives has allowed them to transform their differences into assets. The skills and strategies they developed at university continued to work for them in managing the new challenges they encountered. All of them have found their share of the good things that life has to offer in the world beyond university. They are thoughtful, self-aware and talented self-advocates.

If you look at the lives of these six individuals with a researcher's eye, what do you see? All of our contributors are high achievers and continued to use education in post-secondary programs to further their careers. They earned university degrees at the Bachelor's level and added a second degree to provide a professional credential. Four of them have also completed Master's degrees.

In addition to their educational successes, all six have ongoing employment in professional careers. They drew on talents and interests they had developed as young people outside of school to build a foundation for their careers. They are self-supporting and have homes with family and community connections. Four of them are parents and they are actively engaged in finding resources for their children and passing along the strategies for learning that worked for them. All have taken risks and learned from their struggles. They have been able to adjust to changes and take positive steps to deal with the stresses and frustrations in their lives. Creative problem solving and negotiating for necessary accommodations are an automatic response to the barriers they encounter. They still want to learn and they still want to help others. They are both realistic and optimistic about what the future holds. Would these accomplishments meet the criteria established by researchers to define adult success? I think the answer is a resounding yes.

Along with these markers of adult success, their conversations reveal that our contributors are successful in their own eyes. Each one has a different vision of success but they all feel they have made a place for themselves that fits with the goals they hoped to achieve. Looking back at their own progress, they don't deny the hard work of managing the barriers created by their learning styles. They are realistic about the stresses and challenges to their health that dealing with their disabilities brings, but they have not lost their optimism or a belief in their ability to find a way forward. They share a view of operating in the world that allows them to see opportunities rather than feeling defeated by the obstacles that their deficits create. Their lives continue to be filled with contradictions and surprises but they have put the doubts of others behind them and believe their success can continue.

These six individuals really have surpassed the expectations that most people had for their future. Coming to university looked like a big risk, but it turned out to be the start of their success in finding a place in the adult world. Think of John, who has trouble following a shopping list or finding his way home in a new environment. Now he leads the way through complex problem-solving sessions for multi-national businesses. Then there is Bob, who is a university librarian happily surrounded by books, helping people find research resources he would struggle to read himself. His high school friends would be surprised that he was anywhere near a library or a university. When Jay was young, he had to be forced to go to school and now he is a teacher. He struggles to make his own notes but he has written more than one thesis and authored many successful grant applications to find adaptive technology for his students. Chris is defeated by the thought of reading storybooks to his children, but running a social service agency or a national advocacy network fits him just fine. Sophie isn't a big reader but she takes time to show her children the fun of listening to audio-books and exploring ways to learn about the world around them. Much of the rest of her time is spent being a multi-tasking educator in her community and running an e-business from her dream house by the sea.

How are these things possible? It isn't easy, but every day our contributors find the answers to that question. You could say that succeeding against the odds has become a habit. The discrepancies in their abilities have provided them with some unique challenges both practical and emotional. At the time of their diagnoses, these successes seemed unlikely. But they have all figured out how to do things that might seem impossible at first glance. They may have stumbled but they all continue to routinely achieve in ways that should make us all take a second look at what is possible. As Sophie told a dyslexic student, "Yes you *can*! You just have to figure out *how* you can do it."

Figuring it out and coming to terms with a learning disability is no simple matter. Having a learning disability presents a complex problem. Learning is a lifelong process. It doesn't just happen in the classroom or stop when you leave school. Adaptive technology can't solve every problem. Challenges change with age but they do not disappear. As Chris points out, "there are career, social and family aspects to having a learning disability as well as the educational ones, plus the emotional impact and the impact on self-esteem". Part of the secret to the successes we have seen here lies in the ways our contributors have faced that lifelong reality. They balance the difficulties their disabilities present with an array of creative, winning strategies that allow them to express their strengths and be successful contributing adults.

In these pages there is much good news. We have repeatedly seen individuals with learning disabilities get education, find jobs, build careers and excel. They show us it is possible to balance the demands of a home and a family. We see that self-advocacy and negotiating for accommodations can work in education and with employers. Creative strategies and past accomplishments can count in a classroom and in a work place. Even in highly competitive fields, people will hire you if you tell them you have a learning disability. You don't have to stick with the familiar and stay where people know you. You can have choices and opportunities and be welcomed as a valued professional. Some situations may seem unfriendly or indifferent, but they are not necessarily impossible. You can negotiate for accommodations and find working partnerships. There are many environments where teachers or employers and colleagues are comfortable dealing with all kinds of difference As Bob tells us, "Being different is trendy now!"

Lessons Learned

These conversations reveal the diversity of strengths and deficits that come with a learning disability, as well as the wide of range of styles and strategies that can lead to success. Our participants faced different challenges with different resources and they emerged with different solutions. Some of them felt most comfortable socially in the midst of a community that offered many options for accommodations. They could manage a high degree of dependence on others and were very skilled at developing working partnerships. Being flexible and swapping skills to accommodate their disabilities was the best way forward for them. Others preferred settings where they could avoid their deficits or work around them with technology and the use of extra time. Sometimes their mixed history of success has freed them up to persevere and to take risks that others might not. Gradual progress with careful planning and goal setting keeps others comfortable enough to succeed. As Jay points out, "There is no single magic solution." Difference is at the heart of a learning disability and that is another part of the challenge.

Although there is not one clear route for people to follow, we have seen that there are common themes in achieving success as independent adults. My role, working with these six people at university, was to help them build the new skills and strategies they needed to reach their goals. Self-awareness, self-acceptance and self-advocacy were at the heart of our discussions. Learning to assess courses and environments for optimal opportunities, and negotiating needed accommodations, were frequent topics. Together we looked for ways that they could play to their strengths as learners and minimize the impact of their deficits. Paired with this was the discussion of feedback from both successes and failures. This allowed for improving strategies or revising goals. The students took responsibility in this process and led the way. Facilitating a sense of ownership and control was an important element in their success.

University was a good place for these young people to learn and practice using adaptive technologies and alternative techniques for accessing information and demonstrating their knowledge. Every year they had many chances to discuss their disabilities with a variety of people and negotiate for the accommodations they needed. They became effective self-advocates. I wanted them to learn those enabling skills and strategies in a way that would allow them to see opportunities in the midst of any of the problems they might encounter. We were aiming for success in the short-term goals and in the life skills that could be transferred beyond university. Perhaps the critical element in this whole process was the ability of the person with the learning disability to take control of the learning process and as Alice described, "begin to work with a disability not against it".

There were points when their graduation was in doubt but for all of them, the university years ended in triumph. I felt they had earned more than a degree. All of our contributors developed interests and goals that they wanted to pursue. Jay, Bob and Chris used government-funded projects to gain experience as newcomers in the workforce. These programs helped them establish their success credentials as employees. John, Alice and Sophie used the skills they had demonstrated in sports, extra-curricular activities and summer employment in building their careers. Since they had all learned how to be successful in formal educational settings, they could add professional credentials as well as more practical experience to their resumés. Learning to highlight their abilities and comfortably discuss accommodations for their deficits has served them well in job interviews. They weren't always the successful candidate but with time, persistence and experimentation, they have found workplace environments where they can express their skills and settle into satisfying careers.

Hard work and determination are among the qualities that most successful people will tell you are keys to their success. It certainly was part of how our contributors mastered the effective skills and strategies that are now automatic for them. But these conversations have shown us that hard work alone is not enough. Flexibility and creative problem-solving are needed. When you have a learning disability you often cannot do what is required in the same time or in the same way as others, no matter how hard you try. This usually becomes painfully and frustratingly obvious in the early years at school. Too often effort becomes the focus of attention rather than failure to find ways to learn. If the child is left alone to learn through trial and error, it will certainly mean that much hard work and determination will be expended, sometimes with little reward.

Our contributors were determined hard workers and they often faced adverse circumstances. But as students, these six would not accept "a nice little pass" for working hard. They wanted to learn and do well and they needed help from people who saw beyond their failures and believed in their abilities. When they found people who understood their learning differences, they had valuable partners and life became easier. These young students came to understand that failure can be part of a process that leads to success. They learned that failure didn't need to be a permanent state as long as you learn from it and carry on. This was a very important life lesson for them and for those supporting them. Their time and energy was not always rewarded but they didn't let failure stop them. They persisted until they found things that worked. Their parents advocated for them, made them do their homework and expected them to get an education. The positive expectations of people around them made it easier to believe in their own success and keep on working. Eventually, even the doubts of others could be used to motivate another try.

All of our contributors were able to establish and maintain relationships with people who taught, mentored and supported them. They were not alone in their struggles. Throughout their education they were able to use these relationships to solve the puzzles of their learning styles. Through them they discovered information about options for accommodations and technology that could help them. They found role models who encouraged them and showed them how they might put all of the pieces of their puzzle together.

Memories of their difficult days and the struggles of finding the way forward still remain. Even though they are now in their forties, they let us in on the ways those emotional echoes from their past can still add to their daily challenges. When Jay looks at his students, he tells us that solving their disability issues is the easiest part of his job. He maintains that it is the baggage of struggling with their difference that provides the greatest challenge to making progress in their studies.

Maintaining confidence, in the face of situations that require you to perform in ways that you know you cannot, is always stressful. Trying anything new is always a risk. It often requires a new round of problem-solving and negotiations. Spotting the naturally occurring supports and building on them can become routine. But the effort to push through in the face of difference can still be challenging and stressful. It takes courage, extra work and determination. Sometimes challenges and change are welcome and the excitement is enjoyable. Other times it can be too much. They have all had to struggle to find support and extra time when there isn't any. The sting of their difference mostly informs good choices but sometimes it is overwhelming. As Chris tells us, "I can make it look easy, but it isn't".

In their forties, our participants feel both the comfort of their experience and the challenges to their health that the stress of difference brings. We have seen that building up histories of success, and having established routines for dealing with new and problematic situations, makes it more possible to tolerate and manage that stress. John gives us a detailed account of the array of positive responses to stress that have now become automatic for him in organizing his days. They have been essential in breaking the negative cycles of behavior that kept him from succeeding. Time management, exercise and healthy diet routines are just some of the options that can balance energy and stress. Good working partnerships and sources of personal support are also effective tools in managing stress and energy levels. Establishing healthy routines and networks of allies and friends are essential strategies. There is a high price for ignoring them.

These conversations have shown us that skills and strategies are important but success isn't just about the abilities and resilience of the individual. Finding an informed and flexible environment makes learning and success more achievable. A classroom or a workplace that is a good match for using your strengths makes it easier to excel and often requires fewer accommodations. Working partnerships ease progress. Whether you are a skilled self-advocate or just beginning to find your share of effective strategies, it makes a difference if you have supporters who believe you can do well and who are willing and able to help you manage the barriers. Throughout these pages we have seen examples of hospitable environments, helpful contacts and reasonable accommodations that made a difference in both educational and employment outcomes. By providing practical and emotional support parents, teachers, mentors and friends, counsellors and colleagues can and do play important roles in success.

Since spotting good matches and establishing good relationships are well-established skills for our contributors, it may not be a surprise that most are now married. They have life-partners who understand and support them in creating a home and family. Only Bob has opted for the "simplicity of the single life." Invariably, relationships with partners involve negotiations. The extra dimension is that their learning disabilities demand attention. The family style for all of them has to be organized to include room for accommodating deficits that can't be changed. John has taken over cooking because he can't follow a list at the grocery store. He has to be "selfish" and insist on doing the things he needs to balance his day or "everything falls apart." In some areas, it may not be within their power to compromise or participate. When children are added to the mix, things become even more complicated. John has concluded that the secrets to keeping things going in the right direction are "clear communication, a sense of humour and enjoying time together."

The demands and responsibilities of parenting have not led our contributors to forget the lessons they learned about success. In fact it is just the opposite. Intuitively, they have followed the same paths to developing success characteristics with their children that we see in their own lives. The children discover that there are many ways to learn. They see lots of books and they can read the print or listen to audio versions. Television can provide print captions to the dialogue on the screen. There is computer time to play educational games and get comfortable with technology. There are smart phones that can talk to you, show you pictures, read to you, spell correctly, and help you organize your day. Curiosity and questions are encouraged. Their children are introduced to activities in the community where they can excel and create networks of friends and support. Being physically active for fun and feeling good is a popular pastime. John is already working on self-advocacy and negotiating skills with his daughter in her beginners swim class.

Looking back to their own childhoods, they realize that as parents they need to be good role models. Sometimes it is hard to get through the day with a cool head and patience but they all remember how hard the life of a child can be, with or without a learning disability. All of them stressed the importance of being encouraging and supportive parents but tough enough to be firm and provide constructive expectations and opportunities. They are keenly aware of the genetic links for learning disabilities. When their children behave 'just like me', they are on the alert for further signs of learning difficulties and ready to look for resources and support. Only Chris talks about his fear that his children might have learning disabilities. The pain and sense of isolation from his own youth still haunts him and he does not want to pass that along to his children.

If these young children do have learning disabilities, they will enter a different world than their parents did. They will have the benefit of adults with an understanding of their situation and a home team well-educated in the ways of managing a difference. Advances in technology are changing the world for everyone and in the process they are providing more readily available enabling alternatives for people with learning disabilities. All of our participants have commented on the increased acceptance and awareness of difference that they have noticed in their own adult lives. Their children will also have the benefit of the progress that educators have made in developing options and programs for their support. Sophie's eldest child is in his first year at school and he is already participating in an intensive literacy program as part of his school day. She didn't have to fight to find it. She is impressed with his progress and relieved to have the support of the school. The difference between this experience and her own illustrates some of the dramatic improvements that have been won. This climate of cooperation between family and schools will allow parents to be partners in minimizing frustration and hurt for everyone.

All of our contributors are supporters of early intervention, whether they are parents or not. They do not want children to struggle through their early years in school the way they did. When they describe the costs, it is hard to disagree. As John points out, everyone is trying to adjust to learning in school when they start. Why not begin taking a look at learning strengths and differences then? Teachers can offer productive alternatives to destructive patterns of behaviour. The sooner it becomes a habit to deal with the challenges that school presents, the better it is for everyone. As we have heard from Sophie and Jay, early intervention programs are now regular features in many schools and communities. These positive approaches combined with the increased awareness and acceptance of difference are reassuring signs that progress has been made.

It seems that our contributors do not have the same sense of urgency about services and programs for adults outside of educational systems as they do for early interventions. At the same time, they recognize that many of their own struggles are still related to their learning disabilities. The challenges of their differences remain and show themselves in their daily lives. New situations always require negotiations. Revealing their disabilities may pave the way to success or to misunderstanding and negative outcomes. Unfair treatment in employment might violate workplace policy or human rights legislation. Career, family, health or financial changes might call for counselling and support where knowledge of learning disabilities would be valuable. Although they are not lobbying for specialized services, they are aware of their own vulnerabilities and curious about the strategies, progress and well-being of their fellows.

Disclosing a disability is never a simple matter, but the extent of the caution they expressed surprised me. At university, talking about their disability led the way to much success. Clearly, the workplace and the wider world seems a less benign and predictable environment. Both personal and economic costs may stand in the way. As Chris and John point out, their responsibilities have increased and "the stakes are higher." Although knowledge and attitudes have improved in general, the stigma still remains and sometimes so does the frustration and impatience. Negotiating for accommodations and educating others can seem like an overwhelming and endless task. Not everyone is aware that success in solving the issues of difference is a valuable credential for employment and an excellent quality in a colleague and friend. Fortunately for the rest of us, the way these six go about their daily lives helps educate others about the possibilities for success.

Looking Back Today

The students I met twenty years ago are now successful independent adults. I still see echoes of their younger selves. Their creativity and their resilience are expressed in the paths they have chosen. The years after university have deepened their understanding of their learning disability and its impact beyond the classroom. I can also see that having a learning disability is not foremost in their sense of themselves anymore. They are neither isolated nor defined by their different learning styles. There are many facets to their identities now. Life has shown them that everyone has problems and issues to work around. At the same time, being a person with a learning disability still makes a difference in their lives. The traces of pain and stress that a difference carries are still present but they have accepted the realities of having a lifelong disability. It may take strength and courage every day to find a way to participate but they don't feel unable to accomplish their goals. Their strategies for success are automatic and just part of how they do things. Like learning differently, finding success is a lifetime process and they have found their way to move forward.

We had all hoped that their successes at university, the strategies they developed and the ability to see themselves as able participants would equip them for the lifelong challenges their differences impose. Now time has shown that it has! Seeing themselves with a practical acceptance of both strengths and weaknesses is a way of being in the world that frees them up to be creative problem solvers and contributing, independent adults. Accepting and dealing with their disabilities has allowed them to transform their differences into assets for success. Whatever their choices, all of our contributors have been able to develop and market their strengths, and use their negotiating skills to get the supports they needed. Being a self-aware, self-accepting and creative self-advocate is a worthy goal for anyone but this played an essential role in the successes we see here.

These six individuals have independently made good use their self-advocacy skills and creative problem-solving abilities to build successful adult lives. But Chris asks, "If I had not learned those skills at university, where would I have learned them?" This is a very important question. Parents can model problem-solving strategies and create opportunities to develop special interests and talents that build self-awareness and confidence outside of the classroom. They can encourage independence and help build life skills and social networks. In partnership with educators, this picture can look much brighter. The challenge falls to educators and service providers to take action and provide opportunities to introduce these enabling skills earlier into the lives of their students.

It is important to recognize that success strategies can be developed at any age. Awareness of the possibilities and supports for people with learning disabilities has led more adults to come forward for assessment and assistance. They may have slipped through the schools of their youth unaware of ways to manage their difference but it is not too late for them to discover new skills and strategies. Bob Macdonald might have remained working at minimum wage jobs if he had not come forward after high school and found the strategies for success. This allowed him to cope with the demands of further formal education and build a career he enjoys. Post-secondary education and training programs can be ideal environments for developing success strategies and unlocking the barriers to satisfying careers. Informed programs can offer credentials and skills to adults with learning disabilities that open doors to careers and salaries that match their abilities and interests. Underachievement does not need to be the theme of their stories.

Success in education and in employment is not only a reasonable expectation but a reality for people with learning disabilities. Their paths may have been different but all of our contributors have found that there are many ways to learn and many ways to participate and to excel. The barriers they have faced may have seemed insurmountable but we have seen that this was not the case. Importantly, I know from the many students who come back to visit that these six people are not alone in their success or in their desire to be a contributing part of an informed and welcoming public. Promoting accessibility and awareness in communities and in workplaces can facilitate success for people with learning disabilities. Fueled by their participation, a stronger, more vibrant place to work and learn is created. We saw this happen at our university. Now you have seen some of the many ways it can happen. We hope you will spread the word and make success a possibility wherever you can.

13
Developing Success Strategies

It has been well over twenty years since I began working in a university setting. I am cheered by the progress that has been made in understanding and supporting success for people with learning disabilities. Today, the richness that diversity affords is widely acknowledged and debated. Both the advantages and the difficulties of dealing with difference are now topics of general discussion. But the reality is that vulnerable learners and their supporters will always have to face barriers that individual differences impose. In my time as a counsellor, I have seen that overcoming obstacles can create resilience and turn difference into an asset. These conversations have strengthened my belief that lessons learned and skills built in an educational setting can be life skills that work in the wider world beyond the classroom. Some factors stand out in the successful management of learning disabilities. The ability to take control and become an effective self-advocate is critical. Establishing and maintaining good working partnerships, and finding or creating environments that highlight strengths, all played a role. Now we have seen that this is true for both education and employment.

Self-awareness and self-acceptance are the stepping stones to mastering those skills. They work best when they are an integrated part of a world view that values difference, creative problem solving, hard work and flexibility. Creating that environment for living and learning can begin at a very young age and can be beneficial at any age. Our contributors have found many ways to learn and to succeed and they are showing the young people in their lives how to do it too. Seeing solutions beyond barriers makes learning and success possible. The sooner people with learning disabilities come to understand their learning style and how to accommodate their deficits, the better it is for everyone.

These conversations also show the importance of continuing to educate others about the ways that environments can become welcoming and supportive. Finding ways to succeed should not depend on the resilience and ingenuity of the individual alone. Learning and working environments can be part of the problem or part of the solutions. Our contributors have given us examples of working and learning situations that facilitate their success and some that do not. We have seen how a climate of informed and flexible cooperation allows the expressions of talents and creativity. Educated goodwill and working partnership can ease the way to success. There are hospitable environments where teachers and employers and colleagues expect to be dealing with difference and value it. We need to create more environments like that.

In these final chapters we take a closer look at the process of developing success strategies and welcoming environments from my point of view as a counsellor. The successes of these contributors and their thoughtful reflections speak to the enduring positive effects that education can have on the lives of students. As forty-year-olds, they are still enthusiastic about the lessons they learned at university and the support they received. They continue to use those strategies and pass them along to others facing similar challenges. Their obvious success is an important endorsement for the program of support that we developed and I think the lessons we learned together still ring true. Educating students and building educated environments are a winning combination. Our program was designed for a post-secondary educational setting but it could also be adapted for use with different ages and in other learning situations for adults.

Building Skills for Success at University
Some people leave high school ready to take on the responsibility of managing their learning style but many students with learning disabilities come to university or enter the workforce unprepared. They often have little experience negotiating for their learning needs and developing the learning partnerships that will lead to their success. They may leave high school with only a vague understanding of their learning strengths and weaknesses and a marked sense of discomfort in talking about them. This presents a formidable barrier. A basic understanding of learning strengths and weaknesses is needed to plan and accommodate effectively. Developing this understanding can begin at an early age with a simple discussion of learning strategies that work or don't work in day-to-day routines. The shape and language of these discussions changes as a child matures. With time, experience and good feedback individuals can develop many levels of awareness and acceptance of their learning disability. There is no denying that self-awareness and understanding of learning disabilities appear repeatedly in lists of variables associated with success in both education and employment. Importantly, they are the foundation of effective self-advocacy.

It is sometimes difficult to obtain a detailed individual learning profile and a clinical diagnosis of learning difficulties. Many parents have wrestled with this problem since it is often a critical part of getting institutional support and accommodations. Post-secondary systems usually require students with learning disabilities to bring their psychoeducational assessments with them in order to qualify for support services. Students often regard their reports as secret and potentially threatening. They can be mystifying documents, but they can also be an important part of building understanding and control of a learning disability for the students and for those assisting them.

The majority of students that I encountered as they entered university did not understand or value the information in their assessment. Many had never gone through the process of reviewing their own reports with someone who could explain the findings and discuss their implications. If they had, they felt too uncomfortable to ask the questions that would allow them to understand the contents. Students were usually intensely curious about their results, although they might be ready to reject the findings and their usefulness.

Once the psychometric language was translated, most students found the information about their learning strengths and weaknesses to be immensely helpful. Matching the findings with their own experiences was a way of understanding the puzzle of their learning pattern. Finding both a vocabulary and a safe, interested audience to discuss learning was usually a huge relief, or at the very least a place to begin. It allowed them to build both awareness and communication skills. It also became clear to them that there was a rationale for confidence in their abilities. They realized that they did not have to rely on blind faith, charity or perseverance alone to get them through. They could see and discuss the qualities that made them good candidates for university and a future career.

In discussing the learning strengths and weaknesses revealed by their assessments, we tried to make links with past experiences and current learning situations. Since I did not know them and they did not know what university offered, this was good common ground for developing a working partnership. We exchanged ideas about learning disabilities in general, and efforts at remediation and education. Sometimes this information had a visible emotional effect on the students and provided an opportunity to express some of the concerns that had defeated their hopes of success.

After sorting through the implications and recommendations of their reports, things began making more sense, both to me and to the students. Often patterns of behavior that had seemed unrelated, both inside and outside of the classroom, began to fit together. Exploring the details of their assessments allowed the students to develop ways of understanding and talking about their learning style. It provided them with a framework that integrated both their strengths and weaknesses, and gave them options to consider for accommodating their disability. They could find ways of using their strengths and minimizing their weaknesses. This was an important step in helping them take control of their new learning situations.

A necessary part of the development of self-awareness is learning to find sources of feedback and using them effectively. This is not easy for people with learning disabilities. By definition, information processing presents difficulties. Their learning differences also mean that much common wisdom and standard instruction does not apply to them. Students with learning disabilities have put many extra hours into special programs that have still left them unable to master skills that most people take for granted. They receive many negative messages from their failure in deficit areas.

Often grades on tests do not reflect either effort or knowledge, only lack of effective accommodation. Some tasks are almost effortless while other things are seemingly impossible. The amount of time and effort expended cannot always be a guide, since it is not necessarily connected with results. Their mixed pattern of abilities adds further confusion. Many of the usual sources of feedback simply don't work for them. In order to carry on, students with learning disabilities have to learn to shut out many of the messages that are routinely directed their way. I am sure that if the students I saw had not blocked out a great deal of the feedback they had received, they would not have arrived or continued at university. It is easy to see how a person could begin to rely on luck, charm or passive acceptance in order to cope.

However, as useful as it may have been at times, ignoring feedback can get you into a lot of trouble, both socially and academically. Figuring out a functional system to guide your behaviour is essential. Students tell me that it can seem a bit like trying to crack a secret code. This difficulty with using feedback may be one of the reasons that mentoring and learning partnerships are so vital for students with learning disabilities. Someone who enables them to understand and use the messages they receive, is a valuable lifeline. Students will often tell me about teachers, parents or friends who could understand them and translate the messages from the world around them in ways that made sense to them. These experiences marked the beginnings of the working partnerships that were essential in helping them find their way through school. Regrettably, these mentors often stood out as treasured exceptions rather than the general rule.

Succeeding at university requires effective learning partnerships with a variety of people. The list can include professors, classmates, other students with learning disabilities, librarians, tutors, mentors and counsellors. There are many people who can become sources of feedback and support in managing the learning environment at university. With most of the students I saw, discussing the meaning of feedback from learning strategies, learning partners and social situations occupied much of our counselling time. We would look at their experiences together and try out various possibilities of cause and effect. We would move from there to solving problems, learning from mistakes and enjoying success.

Students could come to the Counselling Centre to refocus and organize their plans during weekly appointments, or when they ran into problems. Our approach was always to assess the situation and then look for ways to maximize strengths and minimize the impact of weaknesses. The next step was to set some goals, pick some strategies, make the necessary adjustments and see how they worked. In time, this process became their own. Learning was not viewed as a binary process of win or lose. Their assessments and their previous accomplishments vouched for their abilities. Tests and assignments were simply seen as a way of getting feedback to adjust strategies. Exams did not prove whether they were smart or dumb. A failed assignment did not mean that they should not be at university. It was a signal to get some more information and make some changes. With guided practice this way of looking at themselves and their learning environment could become automatic and a big part of the crippling fear of evaluation and failure could then disappear.

Once students believed that learning was an ongoing process that could be discussed and managed, they were well along the path to success. This way of looking at the world made them less vulnerable to the barriers that their disabilities created. Reframing the picture, both of themselves and their learning environment, gave them greater chances for success. They were freed up to look for opportunities to learn in the ways that they learned best. Their energies could be directed towards negotiating for the accommodations they required to move forward toward their goals.

Negotiating effective working partnerships is a valuable life skill. It begins with being able to introduce yourself, talk about your learning situation and offer some possible options for accommodation. Once a foundation of self-awareness and accommodation strategies has been established, that may sound like a pretty straightforward set of tasks, but disclosing a learning disability is rarely straightforward. It is an issue which can be tangled with many other sore points. Self-confidence, self-acceptance and previous negative experiences all play a role. Compounding the problem is usually a simple lack of information and an absence of practice. Establishing a partnership with a counsellor, where you can rely on confidentiality and professional experience to get you through the awkward bits, provides an excellent practice ground for branching out to tougher audiences.

Speaking to professors and peers is fraught with concerns about power and prestige. Who really needs to know? When and how should the first contact be made? These are questions with many answers. Levels of comfort, necessity and preference vary widely. Reviewing the options and the costs, and then allowing the student to exercise control over these approaches makes an important statement about responsibility and respect for the student's wishes.

In my experience, students try a variety of approaches to establish working partnerships with their professors. These range from requesting an official letter of introduction from the disabilities program at the start of the year, to making a last minute e-mail or phone call just before a test or a deadline (not recommended). Sometimes a three-party meeting took place with the counsellor facilitating. Eventually most students settle into an independent routine which they have cobbled together from suggestions by peers, practice sessions and previous attempts. The first contacts are the most difficult, but trying to hide a learning disability takes a tremendous amount of energy and ignoring it is usually disastrous. Even the most awkward of approaches may become helpful. The student's willingness to actively engage in managing the learning process is the ingredient that is essential for lasting success. The most important element is simply to get started.

Once a dialogue has begun, ways of getting feedback and assistance from the professors can emerge as the communication develops. Early approaches to professors and support services usually make the process run more smoothly. When people are shown the thought and organization that is involved in managing a learning disability, they are more easily enlisted as allies. Some experienced students interview their professors and review course outlines with them before they enrol. The details of accommodation can be agreed upon and taped texts can be ordered, or readings begun over the summer term. This way, the stressful initiation of a new learning partnership has already been handled, and the student has begun the contact by demonstrating a high level of motivation and maturity. This advanced preparation is very helpful to senior students, but it is a strategy that most first year students would find unthinkable. The more informed and confident the students become about their learning styles, the easier it is to initiate and maintain contact with professors. The more informed the professors become about learning disabilities, the easier it gets as well.

Cautionary Comments

Some students cannot take the steps I have just outlined. Other students are already capable negotiators and advocates. They need only to work out the adjustments necessary for their new environment. Patterns vary. Students with disabilities view specialized support services in a variety of ways too. Some students use transition programs and begin planning before they have been accepted into the university. Other students believe the farther they can stay away from disability services the better their lives will be. Failing or receiving an academic penalty forces some students to identify their disability. Becoming successful and needing to get the best marks possible to go on to further education brings other students to the program. Some students will come for counselling, but do not want to identify themselves to their professors, or take any accommodation that would declare their situation to their classmates. Sometimes professors spot talented students whose hard work is not matched by the grades they receive and refer them along. Some students come because their parents insist, or a friend who knows convinces them it is a good idea. Some students take a look at what is involved and would rather fail or leave.

Students find their way to support at different times and in different ways. A university community aware of disability issues allows students many sources of support beyond the designated special services. The student's willingness to receive support is an important consideration. The principle of accommodating difference has to be modelled by the support service. Sometimes it is painful to watch students making choices about the kind of accommodations they will accept and use, but it can be part of a developmental process for the student, especially if the support program can assist them in reframing and reorganizing their approach when the time is right.

I have learned how important timing is for effective intervention. Strategies that seem too risky to try at some times are easy for students to implement at others. Sometimes failure makes them bold enough to try, or success makes them confident enough to experiment. Standard calculations for reasonable accommodations and appropriate compensation techniques are helpful guidelines, but timing, context and the student's level of comfort and confidence are major factors to consider in developing a workable learning plan. Systems and institutions press for uniformity. I think it is very important that the services for people with disabilities do not fall into the same trap. Maintaining a connection with individual students and allowing them to set their own path and pace has been a big part of our success.

Since you have read the stories of some of these students, you will know that what I have described in a few pages is not a simple process. Students with learning disabilities face a difficult balancing act. They must acknowledge both the internal and external barriers and the strengths they possess to move beyond them. They must recognize and create opportunities for success even when these are not obvious to others. This involves courage, patience and hard work, but these are qualities which are available to anyone. They can be modelled and nurtured at home, in the community and at school, no matter what the strengths and weaknesses of a learning profile are.

Understanding who you are and who you want to be, as a person and as a learner, absorbs a great deal of energy for most young adults. It is a gradual process which unfolds with experience. Self-awareness and self-acceptance are not easy goals, but they are worth the struggle. They are appropriate goals for every student, but they are complicated by the facts of being learning disabled. How do I learn best? How can I show what I have learned? How different does my disability make me? These are critical questions for students with learning disabilities to re-examine as they become adults. University can be a good place for them to explore these questions and push the boundaries of their abilities for an answer. Professors, role models, mentors, parents and counsellors, all can play an important part in helping them find the answers.

Programming for Success

Learning to succeed at university is a developmental process for all students and it involves the whole of the community. Ideally, there is a program and policy of support in place to help with this process for students with disabilities. Here is a look at the structure we adopted to facilitate the development of success strategies for students with learning disabilities.

Prospective students would have some transition visits to the campus before they arrive to start their first term. It is not a requirement for anyone but it certainly is helpful when it is possible. A visit to our resource room is included as part of every high school tour. Individual meetings are a favoured option to discuss services and course selection. Sometimes a parent or teacher comes along to add their support. At registration time, students with disabilities participate in the general orientation process for the university. In addition, our program creates social and workshop opportunities for new students to meet other students with learning disabilities.

First year students have the choice of starting the year with weekly individual meetings in our office. Emergency visits or drop-in meetings are available. Quick access is an important option. It provides an excellent opportunity to model crisis management, or advocacy and conflict resolution techniques. With a supportive listener, students can unpack the elements of their problem and the emotions involved. Whatever form the contact takes, it gives students the chance to examine their beliefs about themselves and their learning strategies in a new light. They can regroup and reframe their situation. Gradually they begin to use these management techniques for themselves.

Working partnerships may need to be developed with note takers and tutors and fellow students in general. We have lists of volunteers available but usually the best partners are found by the students themselves. The major challenge is developing a good working relationship with professors. One of the best ways we found for us to facilitate these working partnerships was to take an active role in offering supervised examination settings and letters confirming the legitimacy of requests for accommodations. One of our staff members coordinates the provision of rooms and proctors for adjusted exams, and supports the negotiation process for both students and professors. Using the exam service provides an opportunity for discussions of reasonable accommodations and learning strategies. The students must begin the dialogue with their professors to set the service in motion. Having an exam service makes it easier for students to request exam adjustments and easier for professors to agree. The students do not feel they are asking for extra favours and the professors are not left to improvise appropriate alternate conditions for the students. Both the professors and the students get to meet others who are using the service. Everyone has the security of knowing that there is a university system to back up their individual needs and that they are not alone in using it.

The first two years are usually the times of most frequent visits to the center. As skills and confidence develop, most students move toward less contact until it is time to begin planning for graduation and the next step forward. Planning for the transition out of university is easily as difficult as planning the transition in. Keeping up with the demands of their current programs usually leaves students little time and energy for considering career options and making applications for employment or further studies. In addition to assisting students in using the career resources available on campus, we provide opportunities for students to attend panel presentations with employers or meetings with alumni mentors where issues of disclosure and workplace accommodation can be discussed along with the usual job hunting or graduate school concerns.

We also encourage senior students to participate in our Speakers' Bureau. Acting as panelists and educators provides leadership experience along with a sense of personal progress. The contacts and confidence developed in this way are often useful in finding job opportunities, and in building interview and resume skills. The students inevitably receive encouragement from their audiences and a sense that their struggles will make a difference for others.

In spite of the hectic pace of the final year, we always try to create opportunities for the senior students to look back over their time at university and reflect on their experience with both peers and supporters. This process is useful for them and a valuable source of feedback for our program. These activities contribute to the resilience and resources that will be needed to face the challenges of a new environment. Sometimes a necessary adjustment is simply to take extra time. I have seen students put to good use a year of further studies at university, work placement programs, volunteer experience or travel. A change of scene or a more relaxed pace can be a very helpful accommodation.

Looking Back

I realize that listening to the students, and trying to support them in finding effective strategies, was exactly the right thing to do. Since there were no well-worn paths to success or teams of waiting experts, the individual students took the lead and assumed responsibility. I did not know the best thing for them to do. Maybe the way forward was not clear to them either, but we tried to sort it out together. I introduced them to accommodation strategies and models of success. We would make a plan and if it did not work out, I would be there to help them pick up the pieces. We found ways of making the existing structures of support work in spite of learning differences. We had to focus on accommodation and compensation techniques, and use the resources at hand to the best advantage possible. That was our agreement. In the process they learned to highlight their strengths and be effective self-advocates who could negotiate for the conditions they needed to be successful.

There was a mutuality in that process that I hope remains fundamental to the way programs operate today. It implies a confidence in the students that acknowledges their abilities, their independence and their previous success. It gives them ownership and control in a way that goes to the heart of the developmental hurdles young people face at university. It allows these students to develop the confidence and skills around their disability issues that they need to carry forward into their adult lives. When this happens, we have seen the success that follows.

Another Cautionary Comment

Today at the post-secondary level, many options are available to people with learning disabilities. It is standard practice to have a program and policy of support that includes access to exam accommodation, adaptive technology and a counsellor. As participation of students with learning disabilities grows, my concern for current programming is that the focus on individual differences will be lost and operating in partnership with students as we see above will be neglected or abandoned. Sending a letter of request from a program office for policy compliance regarding accommodation and setting up adaptive technology is an important start. But it doesn't address the multitude of other factors that make university a success experience. Critically, it does not begin student engagement as a responsible adult partner in learning and achievement.

Even though starting the personal contact with professors might be stressful for students, all of our contributors agree that having that responsibility was an invaluable part of their progress. Guided practice in a relatively benign and consenting environment served them well not only in university but later in dealing with getting a job and building a career. More than that, these personal contacts are meaningful ways to educate professors about differential learning.

Through their efforts, the students with disabilities energize and fuel the growth of a flexible and welcoming learning environment around them, as well as building their own strengths and abilities. We see here that this approach worked and the benefits continued beyond university. Teaching effective self-advocacy skills and building the awareness and acceptance that it requires is such an important link to success that it should not be overlooked.

I hope these conversations will encourage more participation by students in shaping their own success. I also hope they promote activism on the part of professionals and supporters to insist on programming that develops self-awareness, self-acceptance and self-advocacy for all ages. Without these elements the skills, strategies and technology lose their guiding purpose and much of their power.

14
Community Education and a Program of Support

In these conversations we have seen that students with disabilities and their allies went a long way in educating others about learning disabilities. By being effective self-advocates in their daily lives the students not only developed critical skills for their own futures, they also increased awareness throughout the community. They were role models for their peers and good examples of success strategies. Fellow students, their note takers and tutors, professors, librarians and the host of people they encountered on campus learned how to make good working partnerships with people who needed to do things differently. There were private and public discussions to create informed good will. Our Speakers Bureau was busy making the community aware of the successes of students with disabilities and lobbying for supports and policy to back them up. Surely this can happen in employment environments and the wider world too. Out of necessity we made use of the naturally occurring supports and broadened their ability to be effective resources for all students.

At university, these students were resilient but vulnerable learners who needed an informed and cooperative environment to thrive. The same could be said for new employees in the workplace. It is important to know that you don't need to be an expert to start working toward building an environment of educated goodwill that supports learning and success in its various forms. It just takes a few willing hands to get things started. Educating ourselves, our workplaces and our communities is worth the effort.

To encourage you to take action, we offer a template from our experiences. Here are the steps we took together to build a program of support and to educate the community about creating an environment that facilitates the success of people who learn differently. It has now been more than a decade since I left the program described here but I believe the lessons we learned still ring true. Informed educators, employers and colleagues provide opportunities and critical support to help make the links between disability and success a reality.

Students with Learning Disabilities: Clients and Educators
My job as a counsellor in student services at the university gave me the opportunity to meet a variety of students, both inside the counselling office and outside as an educator for residence staff and

other campus groups. This was how I began meeting students with learning disabilities. Some of these students were thriving in the university environment and held high profile leadership positions. Others came to see me because the stress of coping was overwhelming and they needed support. The issues these students struggled with were familiar to me in theory but my past experience involved diagnosis and research with young children. These students knew more than I did about being at university with a learning disability.

What I did know was that all of these students must be very capable people. They must have had many strengths as well as a strong commitment to their educational goals or they would not have found their way to university. I believed in their abilities and in the power of the environment either to shut them out or to facilitate their success. I could see that there were some problems in getting recognition and accommodation for their learning differences. Several students with learning disabilities were very adept verbally, but felt quite defeated when it came to written exams. Sometimes they were able to negotiate alternate forms of testing, but they always felt at the mercy of the professor. If goodwill and understanding were not available, they were stuck.

Many of the students I met had learned very effective ways of assessing and developing goodwill in professors. They were shrewd about course selection, considering both the professor and the types of testing and assignments. They had developed networks of support among their fellow students, their professors and the members of the campus staff. They often showed a high degree of ingenuity and creativity in finding the resources they needed to succeed. Notes, tutors, typists and readers were all part of the resources they needed. Sometimes a kind of skill exchange principle was used. For example, a good set of notes might be exchanged for tutoring, or time on a computer might be bartered for typing services.

Unfortunately, not all of the students with disabilities had these skills, especially not at the start of their university career. Sometimes the informal friendship networks were not available, or sometimes they were not enough. Sometimes goodwill was not available either. Where could these students go for support and advocacy? As in many Canadian universities in the 1990s, there was little institutional recognition of the need for policy or procedures or designated special services for students with disabilities. The Counselling Centre was one of the places students came when they ran into problems. In the quiet of the counselling office, we sat together and tried to sort things out.

I soon came to understand the ways in which the university environment can be very liberating for students with learning disabilities. Students can specialize in their areas of strength. There is more choice when selecting courses and teachers. Fewer hours are spent in class and there is more time to study and complete projects in the way and place that best suits the individual. No one is checking notes or homework and insisting that everyone keep the same pace with daily assignments. In today's classes, there might be power point notes or lectures posted on the internet that can be printed before or after class.

Some students with learning disabilities excel outside of the classroom. Many of the students I met were socially skilled and had taught courses, coached or run youth camp programs. They had already mastered independent group living and knew how to follow their own agendas. This gave them a big head start and they fitted easily into leadership roles in residence, on sports teams or in community activities. Participation in university activities automatically opens up a network of potential friends, study partners and note-takers. For some students with learning disabilities, this means that many of their problems disappear simply because of the way their new educational environment is structured.

However, setting an independent course and taking control of your learning situation is not only a luxury at university, it is a necessity. For some students with learning disabilities the wealth of options can be very confusing. This, along with the lack of an imposed daily structure and continuous teacher contact, transforms the learning situation fundamentally. Understanding the new features of the business of being a student can be hampered by processing and time management deficits. Often planning functions have been taken on by a tutor, teacher or parent as part of their supporting role. This can leave students with very little experience in taking an active role in their own learning. Independent living skills may have been put aside in order to survive the daily academic routine. In these respects the move from home, with the absence of familiar supports and routines, can challenge students with learning disabilities in very stressful ways.

Every student experiences excitement and anxiety starting out on a university career, but for these students learning is different and the stress is intensified. Experience has taught them that being different can be a problem, academically and socially. Even though they have secured admission to a university, their learning histories usually contain minefields of near escapes and negative experiences. New situations must be navigated carefully. They know that everyone expects them to be able to read and write well, and participate in courses in the standard way. They also know that they cannot meet those expectations.

On some level there is always a wish to be like everyone else and leave behind the reality of the resource room and their disabling differences. Who wants to have a problem or be a problem? There is a dread of dealing with the constellation of reactions, ranging from surprise to rejection, that will inevitably be triggered once others get to know about their learning style. The challenge of trying to work out solutions to learning and life problems in a setting with few role models is compounded by having a label with a stigma attached. Imagine the courage and fortitude it must take to persist in formal studies.

From my discussions with these students, I found that the simple acts of listening, affirming their abilities and believing in the possibility of success were amazingly powerful tools. Listening to their experiences established a bond of mutual understanding and provided valuable information that could be used to solve the problems that arose. Many of the students had used such mentoring relationships to good effect on their way to university and had found this type of working partnership with professors and people of goodwill at the university when they arrived. If that was the case, we had valuable sources of support already available on the campus and we could develop more.

At the same time, it was very important to the students that I had a basic understanding of learning disabilities. Not everyone did. They needed my counselling skills and problem-solving approaches too, but the fact that their learning situations were not unknown to me was a valuable part of our connection. The more informed both partners were about learning disabilities, the more effective the working relationships could become.

It seemed obvious that students in this situation would need a support network at university if they were to meet the new demands in their learning environment. They would also require awareness and advocacy from the institution to allow them to participate. The students could change and adjust their own strategies, but if there was no consent or assistance for the adjustments they needed in the classroom and in evaluation, they had some very formidable barriers to overcome.

Educating the Community: Getting Started

Clearly, we needed to build on the positive things that were already happening, but use the existing resources and goodwill in a more informed, accessible and integrated manner. Establishing an organized point of reference for advocacy and information seemed to be the place to begin. For us it was in the Counselling Centre where the first steps were taken. Working along with the students, we began our campaign to educate ourselves and the wider community about the ingredients for success at university for students with learning disabilities.

One of the best resources we had available was the group of students with learning disabilities who were there already. They were teachers for us all. The students who were struggling served to highlight the barriers that existed. The students who were succeeding were excellent role models. The university environment had been a good match for their abilities and they had been able to find ways to minimize the impact of their deficits. They were articulate and engaging young adults who excelled at academics and in community activities. They enjoyed sharing their expertise and telling stories of dealing with resistant professors or surviving time management crises. Perhaps even more helpful were the positive things that had happened in their lives. Their presentations at public forums, seminars and individual meetings allowed us to establish not just the possibility of success for people with learning disabilities, but the reality of it. It became an important part of my role to create opportunities for the exchange of information from these successful students.

Listening to this kind of student expert was a strong motivator for other students with learning disabilities. There was no struggle for rapport or credibility, and there was a wealth of experience and alternatives to discuss. I can still see the looks of surprise and approval on the faces of our new students the day one of our alumni speakers arrived on campus in his new car with his lawyer's suit and laptop. This young man was learning disabled. He was one of them and he had made it. All of the trappings of success were there to prove it. More importantly, he had come to speak to and for them. Once they heard his story they were even more impressed.

Our success marketing campaign began with these young people who had struggled and won. They were very powerful sources of encouragement and insight. They dispelled people's doubts about why students with learning disabilities should be at university. Professors and administrators realized how much we would have lost if these students had been excluded from our community. These sessions helped give students with disabilities a good reputation on our campus and added immeasurably to our network of support. Their presence assisted us in making a space for students with disabilities at the university that was both welcoming and accepting. Some students have told us that our campus was the first place they had ever been where it was okay to be disabled and to be who they were.

To complement these awareness initiatives, I tracked down the leads that the research literature offered. I also sought out colleagues through the Learning Disabilities Association and in other Canadian universities. Service providers from established programs made presentations to our students, teaching faculty and administrators. Student government representatives were keen to lobby around access and disability issues. They put programming and services on the agenda at the university Senate, and at conferences for student union associations at the regional and national levels. Students who were volunteering as note-takers, readers or tutors also took an interest in improving the broader climate of support for their learning partners.

I attended a conference in the United States where a group of researchers reported on models of programming for students with learning disabilities at post-secondary institutions. For me, it was a wonderfully quick orientation to current practice and to the variety of systems available. The cross-cultural aspect was really useful in highlighting common issues in educating people with learning disabilities. Enabling legislation and financing had clearly made a positive impact on services and programming in the U.S., but that was not the only difference to be found. The presentations illustrated a diversity of successful approaches that varied with the size, traditions, resources and strengths of the institutions that used them. I saw how wise it was to tailor program development to the strengths and sources of support that already existed within an institutional structure.

Through all of these investigations, I met some excellent practitioners and made some good friends. I found more good ideas than I was able to implement in over a decade. In adapting these ideas, I was using the same networking and problem-solving strategies that I was advocating for the students. I was able to see first-hand the challenges of locating and using the strategies that fit your own context and strengths.

Some of the students with learning disabilities organized forums and awareness activities for the campus and the community at large. Once this happened, invitations started coming for panel presentations at workshops and conferences. Through our Speakers' Bureau, students were easily contacted for presentations and new students were recruited and coached to participate as educators. The community network of understanding and support expanded.

Educating the University and Formalizing a Policy of Support

Our core of students was highly motivated and had a determination and a commitment to education that was very impressive. As professors met them in classes and as our faculty education and success marketing campaigns prospered, we experienced both the goodwill and the reluctance that existed in the academic community. As in every educational setting, there were some very inhospitable learning environments on our campus. It seemed important to put some formal structures in place to provide institutional recognition and support for students with disabilities. The presence of a policy is reassuring to students and acknowledges that they are expected to be participants in all aspects of the life of the institution. Although a policy does not guarantee fair treatment, it is an important affirmation of commitment and a useful tool for education and conflict resolution.

We turned to our allies within the community to help us build into the system a policy that would both acknowledge the good things that were already happening and make it easier for the students with disabilities to find the resources that they needed. In July of 1990, we formed a Committee for Students with Disabilities. It brought together students, members of faculty, student services personnel and administrators to work toward a formal policy for the university. People with and without disabilities were included. As a group we wanted the institution to offer accessibility and support, but we did not want to promise more than we could deliver. We wanted to keep the student at the center of his or her own learning process, with the university community accepting the responsibility for offering a receptive and cooperative climate for learning.

Because of the small size of our campus population and the many overlapping issues, we decided to work for a policy for all students with disabilities. Our student representatives were adamant that the language used in the program and policy should include the term "disability" so that services and procedures would be visible and immediately recognizable. They felt this was particularly important for new students attempting to find assistance. Their pragmatic frustration over terms like special needs and challenges surprised many of their supporters, but they had their way.

Everyone was well aware that questions of funding could threaten the early acceptance of the disabilities program and policy, especially in the prevailing climate of fiscal restraint. We did not want money to be the stumbling block when so many positive things could happen through recognition of issues of equity and by education on effective strategies of support. We simply wanted to enhance the current structures of support so that they could be a good fit for a broader band of students. We lobbied hard to make these points and our student senators were particularly effective in this campaign.

All of the members of the committee worked together to educate themselves about ways of making university a successful option for students with disabilities. We used all of the professional networks open to us to gather information. The broad base of the committee was extremely useful in this regard. As a group we were able to evolve the necessary consensus for a good policy, just as the larger campus would need to do to implement it.

A policy based on inclusion, self-advocacy and independence seemed to meet all of our needs. In under a year we saw the university Senate unanimously adopt a policy based on our recommendations. The university acknowledged the need to accommodate students with disabilities and to educate the community regarding disability issues. Students with disabilities were welcome to use any of the same resources and services available to every student. Counselling support and accommodation provisions were also available. Choice, control and responsibility for their own success remained with the student. The policy and services were indicated on the admission forms and in the university calendar. Recruiting and publicity materials included similar information.

Over the years, we continued to develop and improve. The Program for Students with Disabilities tried to be a good model of community growth and change. From a small group of informed supporters, we gradually built a broader coalition. Many students with disabilities demonstrated both their competence and leadership abilities. The Committee for Students with Disabilities became a permanent committee of the university Senate, with a mandate to organize and monitor services for persons with disabilities, promote awareness, and develop ways to enable participation of persons with disabilities in the university community. Yearly reports kept the community at large informed of our progress and our plans. We were a regular feature in high school recruitment presentations and in the annual orientation of new faculty. We also took part in residence staff training and panel presentations for student teachers in the education program. Students designed and maintained a disabilities homepage on the university's website. All of these ways of participating indicated that we were a recognized and valued part of the fabric of the university. We took goodwill and turned it into working partnerships.

By 2000, students with learning disabilities made up the largest single group in the Students with Disabilities program. The dozen pioneering students who struggled on their own a decade ago could scarcely believe our numbers. Of course, the program was overworked and underfunded. This is a situation we shared with many of our students and many programs like ours. Not every student who used our program graduated. Some took extra time to complete their degrees, but our statistics were not different from the rest of the campus. Professors appreciated having a resource that they could rely on to sort out reasonable accommodations. Our student evaluations were positive and we had our share of students on the Dean's List for academic excellence. Students with learning disabilities could be found participating in student government, residence staff, varsity teams, media and campus societies. Overall, we created an environment where students with disabilities were expected and welcome.

Inevitably, funding was an issue that would not go away. We had a thin line in the student services budget. To finance our proctoring service for adjusted exams, we relied heavily on a fund established by a group of alumni in memory of a classmate with a disability. Volunteer support was indispensable in keeping many of the services in our program functioning. Note-takers, tutors, typists, readers and aides were often volunteers. We competed for grants and attempted to develop partnerships with other service providers. Together we found funds to improve access for our library system and computer labs.

Intermittently, we received federal government money for support personnel and adaptive technology. Each year we tried to improve physical accessibility on the campus, but we had a long list of improvements to confront. Fortunately, government bursaries are now available to individuals to fund the acquisition of technology and to pay for some of the other extra supports they may require. These programs often seemed hidden behind bundles of paper work and complicated conditions, but with staff support through the details many students do qualify. Access to adaptive technology with training and technical support was still a thorny issue on our agenda. Annual service audits by a committee of students and faculty kept our goals and successes visible.

Our student Speakers' Bureau was very active, meeting with many campus and community groups. They had a regular spot in the teacher training program. Each year we held information sessions on disability issues for the general faculty. The best attendance always came from the sessions where our students invited their own professors. Showing professors the time and creative options that our students used to learn was a very powerful tool. Day tours for junior high students seemed to add an element of hope and encouragement for both the teachers and students at a time when even surviving high school can seem like an unattainable goal. Our transition workshops for senior high school students were important too but they took a large contribution of time and energy. We developed a streamlined version in cooperation with the high school liaison office where high school students with disabilities were paired with a buddy from our program for their day or weekend visit. Many of the students from our program look forward to participating as peer facilitators and mentors in these events.

Students, with and without disabilities, continued to play an active role in the maintenance and the development of the program. Volunteers were our major resources and we needed them. The students with disabilities themselves were our main education agents. They educated their professors and fellow students in the course of their studies and as they presented workshops for community groups. They taught and mentored as they developed and practiced their own skills. I saw a real virtue in this necessity. It insists on an attitude of self-advocacy and independence that is genuine and allows the students to grow in confidence and to own the successes they achieve.

As the Contact Person for Students with Disabilities, I can tell you that the changes we initiated made a difference in day-to-day life on campus. We offered all of the ingredients that the students told us were important. We had a staff person who was informed about disability issues to provide specialized counselling and advocacy services. We had a policy which promoted access and adjustment to mainstream services. We had a person to coordinate the proctoring program for exam accommodations and to facilitate the use of adaptive technology and tutorial assistance. We had an attitude that respected individual difference and a realistic view of the trouble it can cause. Finally, we tried throughout to model a way of looking at the world that allows people to find opportunities in the face of the barriers they encounter.

Our program was not perfect but we were proud of our progress. We felt we were moving in the right direction and the successes of our students showed us this was so. It was still not easy being a student with a disability at university, but we were able to minimize some of the frustrations and provide opportunities for students with disabilities to learn and to excel. All of our students had a chance to learn to negotiate and advocate for their learning needs. These are skills that they can profit from for the rest of their lives. Some of our graduates have chosen careers that allow them to continue to work on disability issues but all of our graduates have a wealth of learning and experience to offer in the communities they join. Educating our community and developing a policy and program of support was a rewarding developmental process for both the students and the institution. Together we found some very good answers to the question of why students with learning disabilities might want to come to university and how an educated community might help them to succeed.

Next Steps

Entering the workforce, changing jobs and developing a career require many of the same steps that we have outlined for dealing with university. Discussions of the issues around disclosure, workplace accommodations and human rights legislation have meant a great deal to people working on resume writing, handling a job interview and matching interests and abilities with a career. The self-advocacy skills and creative strategies of our contributors have served them well but transitions of all sorts often require support. Planning career advances or moving location, fine tuning negotiating skills and anticipating the barriers of any new situation, all might call for an informed resource person. Programs of support that continue across the lifespan would be helpful even to people who are effective self-advocates.

Once adults leave the systems of support provided by educators, it is not always clear how to take the next steps forward. Specialized programming is offered by governments and community groups but access is often limited and complicated with considerations of need, definition and disclosure. On-line sites can help locate resources and provide connections with advocacy groups. Employers, human resources professionals, occupational therapists, vocational counsellors, job coaches and community employment networks can all be possible sources of support, especially if they are informed about learning disabilities. Awareness education, that broadens the reach of these existing services, offers the promise of improving resources throughout the inevitable changes in an adult life. Equally important is to make community and workplace environments more welcoming and accommodating. Participation by people with learning disabilities and their supporters makes a powerful statement about the abilities that go along with a difference. Expecting people with learning disabilities to participate and contribute can become an automatic response that benefits everyone. The experiences of our contributors make it clear that we need to continue awareness campaigns beyond the school room and into all of the environments we inhabit.